Interprofessional **Education for Nurses**

Nurse Education in Practice Series
Interprofessional Post-qualifying Education for Nurses: Working together in health and social care
Edited by Sally Glen and Tony Leiba

Supporting Learning in Nursing Practice: A guide for practitioners
Edited by Sally Glen and Pam Parker

Multi-professional Learning for Nurses: Breaking the boundaries
Edited by Sally Glen and Tony Leiba

Problem-based Learning in Nursing: A new model for a new context?
Edited by Sally Glen and Kay Wilkie

Clinical Skills in Nursing: The return of the practical room?
Edited by Maggie Nicol and Sally Glen

Nurse Education in Practice Series
Series Standing Order
ISBN 0–333–98590–7
(outside North America only)

You can receive future titles in this series as they are published by placing a standing order. Please contact your bookseller or, in the case of difficulty, write to us at the address below with your name and address, the title of the series and the ISBN quoted above.

Customer Services Department, Macmillan Distribution Ltd
Houndmills, Basingstoke, Hampshire RG21 6XS, England

Interprofessional Post-qualifying Education for Nurses

Working together in health and social care

Edited by

Sally Glen

and

Tony Leiba

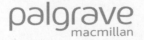

First published 2004 by
PALGRAVE MACMILLAN
Houndmills, Basingstoke, Hampshire RG21 6XS and
175 Fifth Avenue, New York, N.Y. 10010
Companies and representatives throughout the world

PALGRAVE MACMILLAN is the global academic imprint of the Palgrave
Macmillan division of St. Martin's Press, LLC and of Palgrave Macmillan Ltd.
Macmillan® is a registered trademark in the United States, United
Kingdom and other countries. Palgrave is a registered trademark in the
European Union and other countries.

ISBN 1–4039–0516–9 paperback

This book is printed on paper suitable for recycling and made from fully
managed and sustained forest sources.

A catalogue record for this book is available from the British Library.

10 9 8 7 6 5 4 3 2 1
13 12 11 10 09 08 07 06 05 04

Printed in China

Contents

List of Figures   viii

List of Tables   ix

List of Contributors   x

Foreword   xi

Preface   xv

1 Interprofessional Education: The Policy Context   **1**
Sally Glen
   Introduction   1
   The policy context   1
   Conceptual confusion   4
   Ambiguous aims   6
   Implementation: pre- or post-qualification?   8
   Implementation: political, organisational, educational
   and cultural factors   8
   Conclusion   11
   References   12
   Web addresses   15

**2 User and Carer Involvement in Interprofessional
   Post-qualifying Education and Training**   **16**
Tony Leiba
   Introduction   16
   Background   17
   Users' and carers' involvement in education and training   20
   User involvement in research   23
   Facilitating user involvement in education and training   25
   Conclusion   26
   References   27

**3 Work-based Interprofessional Education for
   Community Mental Health Teams**   **29**
Scott Reeves
   Introduction   29
   Background literature   29

Project development   31
Delivering the workshops   31
Evaluation – methodological approach   32
Data collection   33
Data analysis   34
Findings – participating teams   34
Attendance   35
Pre-workshop perspective   35
During the workshops   36
Post-workshop perspective   38
Three-month perspective   39
Discussion   40
Conclusions   42
Acknowledgements   43
References   43

**4   Partnerships in Interprofessional Education and
     Practice: The Development of a Masters
     Programme in Interprofessional Practice   45**
Philippa Sully
Introduction   45
Background   46
Partnership and authority   47
Strategies and structures   49
Triangular relationships   50
Interprofessional practice MSc: society, violence
and practice   51
Student selection   51
Course structure   52
Modules   52
Content delivery   54
Assessment   55
Systems, containment and reflection   55
Programme evaluation   57
Conclusion   58
References   58

5   Interprofessional Practice Teacher Education   61
Dave Sims and Kate Leonard
Introduction   61
The context of practice teacher education   61

Background and development of the course 63
Learning to support learning 64
What is a truly interprofessional course? 65
Uni-professional, multi-professional, interprofessional? 66
Key challenges as the course has developed 68
Feedback from course participants and other stakeholders 71
The views of managers and training officers 73
Impact on professional practice 74
Conclusion 76
Postscript 77
References 77

6 Interprofessional Post-qualifying Education: Team Leadership **79**
Mike Cook
Chapter overview 79
The need for improved leadership 79
Definitions 82
Background to the programme 84
Using the embodying leadership framework to develop a programme 88
How is the programme working in practice? 91
How is learning being assessed? 93
Dedicated web site 94
Support from other experienced leaders 94
A unit of learning described 95
Discussion and conclusions 97
References 99

7 Interprofessional Education: The Evidence Base **102**
Sally Glen
Introduction 102
Establishing the evidence base 103
Work-based interprofessional education 105
Conclusion 106
References 107

Index 108

List of Figures

6.1   Integrated programme structure   90
6.2   Programme outline   92

List of Tables

5.1   Getting the balance right – changes in the student profile   66
5.2   Benefits of being involved in practice teaching   75
6.1   A changing world   81

List of Contributors

Mike Cook, EdD, MSc (Education Management) MSc (Quality Management) DipN (Lond), RN, ILTM
Associate Dean for Learning and Teaching, St Bartholomew School of Nursing and Midwifery, City University, London.

Sally Glen, PhD, MA, RN
Deputy Director of Institute of Health Sciences, Professor of Nursing Education, Dean St Bartholomew School of Nursing and Midwifery, City University, London.

Tony Leiba, PhD, MPhil, MSc, BA, Dip.N, PGCE, RMN, RNT
Senior Research Fellow, North East London Mental Health Trust and the Faculty of Health and Social Care, London South Bank University.

Kate Leonard, BA, MSW, CQSW
Senior Lecturer for Interprofessional Practice Teaching Course, Faculty of Health and Social Care, South Bank University, London.

Scott Reeves, MSc, BSc, PGCE
Research Fellow, St Bartholomew School of Nursing and Midwifery, City University, London.

Dave Sims, MA (Education), BA, DipSW, PGCE
Professional Lead for Social Work, University of Greenwich, London.

Philippa Sully, MSc, Cert Ed, RN, RM, RNT, FPA Cert, CC Relate
Senior Lecturer Interprofessional Practice, St Bartholomew School of Nursing and Midwifery, Institute of Health Sciences, City University, London.

Foreword

I welcome the invitation to introduce this book because deep-down, I do not believe that effective interprofessional team working can be 'taught'. However, this does not mean that it can not happen and therefore, any opportunity to explore issues of interprofessional collaboration are most welcomed, given the challenges it needs to overcome.

To start, I have to declare an interest in the subject in that I have over several years been associated with a number of initiatives both in University and in service settings which have attempted to take forward interprofessional collaboration, with differing degrees of success.

In my PhD supervisor role I have come across case studies of good interprofessional practice, teams that work effectively and where there is respect for each other's professional roles and the contribution each member makes towards the problems or the client's care management and where there is evidence of expert facilitation and leadership at developing relationships between colleagues of different disciplines. Whether this can be replicated at will or whether it is a matter of facilitative leadership and personalities working well together, is what books of this nature may help to describe and evaluate.

In the UK, the interprofessional working agenda has been an aspiration for many years, held by successive governments of different parties, and as stated in the introduction 'resistence to interprofessional education has become politically unacceptable'. A heavy directive indeed, but where is the inducement?

Interprofessional education is burdened with all kinds of difficulties. The book identifies the following:

- Conceptual confusion – confusing/mixing interprofessional with multiprofessional education
- Questions around operationalisation
- The need for systematic review work examining the effects of inter-professional education
- The need to demonstrate the costs–benefits analysis associated with interprofessional education
- Pre- or post-registration implementation?
- Sustaining interprofessional initiatives as well as initiating these.

This book provides five case studies of postgraduate interprofessional education, three of which describe masters level courses involved in inter-professional development, and two which describe evaluative projects involving users and carers participation in education and training and work-based interprofessional collaboration respectively. This is a most welcomed follow-up from the editors' first publication *Multi-professional Learning for Nurses – Breaking the Boundaries* (2002) in which the contributors shared five examples of undergraduate Interprofessional education.

Key areas explored by the various contributors to this book include:

How does interprofessional education impact on professional practice? Should there be an even balance of professionals for a better interprofes-sional experience?

One of the arguments offered is that perhaps attitude and motivation are more important factors together with focusing on a shared service user group, that is, mental health, older people and so on.

It is also identified that within interprofessional courses, requests for uni-professional time to be included should be taken seriously.
The discussion identifies three key outcomes from effective interprofes-sional education which keep recurring in several chapters:

• greater dialogue as different views, values and cultures meet;
• greater understanding as there is increased awareness of professional aspects including roles and responsibilities; and
• evidence of new perspectives arising with increased understanding of different practices in a constantly changing world.

Several authors talk about the importance of ensuring terms are clarified and differences understood. Terms like clinical, mentorship, supervision, have different meanings for different groups.

So, how far does interprofessional working actually improve the services – or not – for the user and carer?
Can interprofessional working close the gaps in service provision from the user viewpoint – the so called seamless care?
Can it bring together all the 'experts' in caring (including welfare workers, volunteers, informal carers and users) in the delivery and use of health and social care.
Does interprofessional collaboration/working increase choice or not? How can user involvement be facilitated in interprofessional education?

How can interprofessional teams integrate more with user self-help groups? An interesting example is given which identifies that the key is in facilitating user involvement in interprofessional education 'by intervening in the group process in the right way at the right time when there is conflict or confusion'.

Interprofessional education does not come cheap. An active investment on people is required if they are to work effectively in partnership across the boundaries of disciplines and levels and become skilled in leading, managing and developing interprofessional and inter-agency collaboration. For example, one of the chapters presents us with an interesting range of interactive teaching methods where two or more experts in the field would jointly teach. Also, module leaders were required to attend their own group supervision. This was included in the programme because of the subject – working with survivors of violence, but it might be also applicable to the successful implementation of interprofessional education in general.

As summarised in the last chapter, when future challenges are discussed, 'Interprofessional education is widely seen as a way to develop collaborative practice among health and social care professions' but:

- What is a successful outcome?
- How is it to be evaluated?
- What is the most effective interprofessional work-based education?
- What characteristics?
- What is the cost? or better still cost–benefit analysis?

Schon (1983) predicted the changing context of professional work when discussing the threats and crisis of confidence in professional knowledge and the trend towards deprofessionalisation. As the tasks/context changes, so will the demands for knowledge. If the hub of professional activity is rigorous problem solving, one way forward would be providing multiple perspectives to this problem solving activity and this involves learning and working together. The challenge though is that interprofessional working is about people getting on well, understanding each other and trusting each others judgement and whether that can be taught or not is a matter of opinion. Nevertheless interprofessional work needs nurturing and examples of good practice.

This book makes a very useful contribution towards the delivery of the government's agenda for an integrated workforce, seamless care and increased user choice, by presenting and evaluating new models of interprofessional teaching and learning but more importantly, in doing so it is not afraid to explore and confront the challenges surrounding interprofessional education.

References

Glen, S and Leiba, T (2002) Multi-professional Learning for Nurses. Breaking the Boundaries. Basingstoke: Palgrave.

Schon, D (1983) The Reflective Practitioner: How Professionals Think in Action, New York: Basic Books, Inc.

Amalia P. Gallego, RN; RNT; MA; MSc

Education Consultant

Visiting lecturer, South Bank University

Preface

In the first chapter Sally Glen contextualises post-qualifying interprofessional education in a socio-political context. The pace of change in health care policy shows no signs of diminishing under the Labour Government. The raft of reforms in health care since 1997 makes interprofessional post-qualification education even more important and possibly more fraught. A significant change under the Labour Government was that education and training are acknowledged as essential factors in enabling the achievement of the Government's aims for health and social care. The delivery of National Service Frameworks, Health Improvement Plans, waiting list targets and the Working Time Directive for Junior Doctors all depend upon workforce design and development. Glen argues that interprofessional education has become overt and managerially driven. Resistance to interprofessional education has become politically unacceptable. Learning together in both the pre-qualifying stage of professional education and subsequently is taken as crucial to opening up the potential for future workforce modernisation.

There is much rhetorical support for user and carer involvement in pre- and post-qualifying education, however Tony Leiba suggests that user and carer views and contributions are often undervalued by educators. Leiba argues that active involvement cannot develop without recognition of the need by educators, and the provision of appropriate preparation for users and carers. He argues work needs to be done to evaluate long-term outcomes such as, understanding the users and carers perspectives and expectations, changes in attitudes, improved communications and that exposure to interprofessional teaching and learning exposure leads to improved care for users.

Acknowledging the seductive nature of work-based learning for managers, Scott Reeves describes a pilot project that offered a series of work-based interprofessional workshops to two community mental health teams. Importantly Reeves' evaluation revealed that heavy workloads inhibited many participants from fully engaging in this type of work-based learning. Given the current drive to maximise the potential opportunities for delivering work-based learning, Reeves argues that further research is required to explore, in depth, the effect of this tension on the processes and outcomes of work-based interprofessional education.

Nationally and internationally governments and service providers are increasingly recognising the extent and consequence of violence. Intentional and unintentional violence includes: domestic rape, torture, suicide, road traffic collisions, transport disasters and violence in institutions and the workplace. Violence causes enormous human costs to individuals, families and society. These issues have raised awareness of the need for interdisciplinary approaches to the care of survivors of violence, as their difficulties can often go unrecognised by health and social care services and employers. Philippa Sully examines the development and implementation of an Interprofessional Master of Science programme for practitioners who work with survivors of intentional and unintentional violence.

Dave Sims and Kate Leonard describe and evaluate a model of interprofessional post-qualifying education developed to meet the learning needs of practice teachers who support students on social work and community nursing qualifying programmes. Sims and Leonard explore the rationale for changing to an interprofessional approach, describe and reflect upon the programme and its development and evaluate the outcomes with reference to an evaluation carried out with former students, their managers and training officers. Key issues which have arisen during the development and implementation of the course are highlighted, in order to identify lessons learned which could be helpful to those developing future programmes of interprofessional education.

The development and implementation of a work-based Interprofessional Masters Degree Programme for staff that lead teams is described by Mike Cook. Enquiry-Based Learning is often used to facilitate interprofessional education. One section of the programme is described in more detail, identifying how the programme participants from diverse areas of health and social care worked in an Enquiry-Based Learning model to explore aspects of 'vision' in leadership.

Evaluations seem to be more sure-footed in capturing students' experience and weighing implications for programme modifications, less so in establishing the impact of learning in practice, still less in establishing the benefit to service users. In the final chapter, Sally Glen argues that given the challenges associated with implementing interprofessional education, it is essential the move is evidence-based. Glen argues that learning together may help people to work together more effectively and is intuitively reasonable. However, this immediately leads to more difficult questions about: For what kind of interprofessional learning experiences should one aim? What are the outcomes of interprofessional education?

How can the impact of interprofessional education be detected? In the context of the prevailing 'evidence-based' agendas, the need to provide empirical support for the value of interprofessional education is increasing. It is vital that research investment is identified and directed towards this policy area. As noted in Chapter 1, interprofessional education has become managerially driven and resistance has become politically unacceptable. Evaluation will be required to legitimate this policy directive.

Sally Glen, City University, London. February 2004
Tony Leiba, South Bank University, London. February 2004

1

Interprofessional Education: The Policy Context

Sally Glen

Introduction

For over 30 years interprofessional education has been evoked as being a means of enlisting joint action across agencies and professions to implement reforms in health and social care. However, the pace of change in healthcare policy shows no sign of diminishing under the Labour Government. The raft of reforms in health care since 1997 makes interprofessional post-qualification education even more important, and possibly more fraught. The delivery of National Service Frameworks, Health Improvement Plans, waiting list targets and the Working Time Directive for Junior Doctors all depend upon workforce design and development (Humphris and Macleod Clark 2002). Interprofessional education seems to be becoming a 'conventional wisdom solution' to a number of concerns arising in relation to professional practice in the NHS (Hale 2002). As a result interprofessional education has become overt and managerially driven. Resistance to interprofessional education has become politically unacceptable. Learning together in both the pre-qualifying stage of professional education and subsequently is taken as crucial to opening up the potential for future workforce modernisation.

The policy context

'The New NHS: Modern, Dependable' (DOH 1997), followed a change in administration after 18 years of conservative government. In the

1

introduction to this document, the Prime Minister states that the change in administration has marked a turning point for the National Health Service (NHS) by the replacement of the 'internal market' with 'integrated care'. Similarly, a further document, 'The NHS Plan' (DOH 2000a) calls for a health and social care system that will be built upon partnership between patients, users, carers and families and NHS staff; between the health and social care sectors; between different government departments and between the public sector, voluntary organisations and the private sector. 'The NHS Plan' (DOH 2000a) provides higher education institutions (HEIs) with many opportunities to extend their relationship with the NHS. 'The NHS Plan' sets out targets and milestones for modernising the workforce and the health service. 'The NHS Plan' also sets out a new agenda highlighting the importance of:

- setting the patient at the centre of the care approach;
- building effective interprofessional team working;
- enabling care to be provided by the staff member with the most appropriate skills regardless of role or title.

'A Health Service of All The Talents' (DOH 2000b) focuses on the systems and culture of NHS workforce planning, in particular, on the rigid differentiation between professional groups, in terms of education and promotion, and also the funding for education. 'The Talents' document suggests that it is the skills and knowledge, which staff can bring to patient care rather than simply their professional background. This document emphasises the service need for new health professional pathways, for example, Public Health Practitioners, Emergency Care Practitioners and Advanced Health Care Practitioners (Cameron 2000).

Healthcare teams in the future are also likely to comprise a greater variety of skill levels. It is inconceivable that the increased demand for health and social care can be met using the current skill mix. The development of Foundation Degrees initiated by the Department for Education and skills, for example, will see the emergence of an 'intermediate professional' in health and social care. These opportunities to provide a different range and level of services will have far-reaching implications for the scope of existing professional territories of practice.

A defining moment in creating a focus for radical change in the NHS has been the Bristol Inquiry into the deaths of children undergoing cardiac surgery at Bristol Royal Infirmary (Kennedy *et al.* 2001). The findings of the Inquiry provided a strong lever for the modernisation of the NHS. The Inquiry brought into stark relief the consequences of professional groups socialised into behaviour patterns and working patterns and working relationships that maintained a pervasive order based on a medical hegemony. The process of socialisation had created a social order of professions which itself became resistant to questioning and change. A diversity of patient and interprofessional perspectives can often open up new possibilities for change. However, the maintenance of the status quo through persistent social norms and values often acts to nullify the sought after advantage of diversity.

From the Bristol Inquiry and the subsequent Department of Health Strategy for lifelong learning (Department of Health 2001), the policy imperative to promote interprofessional and shared learning for health-care practitioners has been significantly advanced (Department of Health 2000, A Health Service of All the Talents: Developing the NHS Workforce: A Framework for Lifelong Learning for the NHS, Department of Health: London 2001). The future preparation of healthcare practitioners should involve developing a better understanding of different perspectives on the same world of health and social care. With this comes the potential for recognition of the respective jurisdictions of practice, developing flexibility, open-mindedness, reducing prejudice and stereotyping, building mutual respect and understanding of the common world of patient centred care. Blurring of role boundaries and recent policy initiatives including the proposed Department of Health's review of the healthcare workforce and proposals outlined in the Agenda for Change document (NHSE 1999), all support the need for radical review of current approaches to educating healthcare professionals.

Between 2000–02 the Department of Health's policy emphasis was on developing interprofessional education within pre-qualifying education. Pragmatic development towards more interprofessional learning is currently taking priority which includes aiming for 'threads' of interprofessional learning in all programmes. Since 2002, the DOH has focused on developing a shared framework for health professional learning beyond registration (DOH 2002a) and linking education to service delivery plans (DOH 2003). There is of course, a need to have a continuation between pre- and post registration education. In the future education programmes for Advanced Practitioners should sit coherently alongside the education programmes required by 'Modernising Medical Careers' (DOH 2002b).

The socio-political 'imperatives' contextualising the above policy documents includes:

- changing health and social care needs;
- blurring of professional boundaries;
- cross sector and cross agency working;
- changing roles and workforce design.

A dramatic shift in the scale of skill mix changes will need to take place if the Government's vision for the NHS and Social Care is to be realised. The key to this vision are the principles of learning together and developing new educational pathways and routes for new role configuration. Successive Governments however have focused more on changing the structures of the NHS than on reforming the working practices, cultures and attitudes of the staff within it (Kendall and Lissaur 2003). Yet these issues are critical in determining the quality of care patients receive. A significant change under the Labour Government was that education and training were acknowledged as essential factors in enabling the achievement of the Government's aims for health and social care. This was demonstrated in the many policies that referred to the importance of education (DOH 1997, 2000a,b, 2001, 2002a,b, 2003). There were three overarching messages within all of these policies which were that, if the NHS modernisation agenda is to be a success, there is a need for, better interprofessional team working, improved recruitment and retention of staff and a workforce that has the appropriate knowledge and skills and is 'fit for purpose'.

Conceptual confusion

'A Health Service of All The Talents' (DOH 2000b) provides a good example of the continuing conceptual confusion that exists in the literature on educational activities that involve two or more different professional groups. A variety of terms have been attached to this activity, for example:

- Multiprofessional
- Multidisciplinary
- Transdisciplinary
- Interprofessional
- Shared learning
- Common learning.

'The Centre for The Advancement of Interprofessional Education' (CAIPE 1997) offers a useful definition of this activity. 'CAIPE' (1997) defines an educational activity that uses *interactive* learning approaches (e.g. small group work between professionals to cultivate collaboration) as 'interprofessional education'. In contrast an educational activity where learning is shared *passively* (e.g. using joint lectures), is viewed as multi-professional education.

Employing CAIPE's definition, it would appear that interprofessional education occupies a low priority in both the HE and NHS agendas. Miller *et al.* (1999) in a research report entitled 'Shared Learning and Clinical Teamwork: New Directions in Education for Multiprofessional Practice', argue that the HE agenda is more focused on promoting multiprofessional education whereby groups of different students for example: medical and nursing students, are offered shared lectures designed to develop their understanding of specific disciplines such as social policy, sociology and ethics. The learning is aimed at providing a common understanding of a subject area, as opposed to, for example, the development of collaborative or team working skills. The latter are of course the key to the effectiveness of post-qualification health and social care professionals within the context of the workplace.

Clearly, there are advantages for employing this type of educational approach. Multiprofessional education is likely to achieve economies of scale and reduce curriculum overlap. However, simply placing students together in large mixed classes can be unproductive (Parsell *et al.* 1998). Students may ignore each other, resent sharing their education with other professional groups or feel that their learning is being 'diluted' (Horsburgh *et al.* 2001). Without the inclusion of interactive activities, this type of educational approach is unlikely to have any impact on enhancing interprofessional collaboration, a central policy aim in this area. Due to this need for student interaction, interprofessional education is by necessity a small group activity (Barr 1996). If students are to benefit from interacting with other professional groups, Barr argues that generous staff–student ratios are required. Interprofessional education puts a premium on innovative approaches to learning and teaching. The emphasis is on individuals learning actively and in collaboration with colleagues from other disciplines – including where appropriate, colleagues from other agencies. However, 'A Health Service of All The Talents' is largely silent in relation to the question of operationalisation.

Ambiguous aims

In response to 'A Health Service of All The Talents' (DOH 2000b), Finch (2000) raised questions about the ambiguity of the documents' aims (Glen 2001). For example, is it for students:

- Know about the roles of other professions?
- Be able to work with others?
- Be able to substitute for others?
- Find flexible career pathways?

Finch (2000) suggests that the above possible ambiguity means that higher education institutions will find it difficult to develop the necessary 'pedagogical approaches' that can underpin this type of activity. In addition, both Finch (2000) and Barr (2000) argue that the proposed role 'substitution' and more flexible career pathways between traditional professional roles will be difficult to implement. Attempts at substitution and flexibility between professional roles are likely to meet resistance given the deeply ingrained professional demarcation lines that exist between NHS staff. Barr (2000) suggests that the introduction of role substitution and flexibility between professional roles creates increased opportunity for interprofessional tension and territorial competition. Barr (1996) thus argues that interprofessional education is primarily focused on understanding and respecting the *differences* between professions. It is not concerned with issues of substitution or producing a flexible, and by implication, a generic health worker. Furthermore, one must not loose sight of uniprofessional education and strengthening individuals' contribution to the team providing care.

The key questions arising from this analysis of the contemporary policy context are:

- Is there a mismatch of expectations?
- Is there a plurality of outcomes required by different stakeholders, which are in tension and contradiction with each other?
- If students learn together, will they be better prepared to work together?
- Can education alone be the sole strategy?

'The NHS Plan' (DOH 2000a), promotes a clear message that better team working and collaboration must be reflected in education if the

NHS is to produce a workforce that is 'fit for purpose' and able to adapt to rapidly changing demands in health and social care. Miller *et al.* (1999) however raises the question:

> In the acute sector, organisational policies have driven working practices towards greater patient throughput by filling as many beds as possible, and staff turnover is high. Despite good intentions ... the development of highly collaborative working practices may be practically impossible ... It is a mistake to think that education alone can achieve better collaborative practice. (Miller *et al.* 1999)

Rigid demarcations and hierarchical relationships have no place in services where boundaries between professions need to be more permeable. As relationships become more flexible, the risk of territorial disputes increases. Therefore, for example, in the case of mental health, efforts to improve collaboration have gone hand-in-hand with those to promote a new model of care. The same has been true in the field of learning disabilities, where staff who were re-deployed from hospitals to the community were retrained and nursing awards were replaced with social care awards (Jay 1979). In these and other fields of community care, for example, palliative care, HIV/AIDS and the care of the frail and elderly in the community, interprofessional education has contributed to efforts to improve the quality of long-term care. It is useful to see the work on interprofessional education as one strand in a series of interlocking initiatives intended to ensure a more flexible and responsive NHS. The initiatives being: job profiling □ workforce planning □ interprofessional education (NHS South West Regional Office 2002).

Although the short-term cost of interprofessional education will inevitably be more expensive than employing a multiprofessional approach, in the longer term, interprofessional education could provide professionals with the necessary skills for effective collaboration and ultimately better quality patient care. However, until there is a firm evidence base for the effects of interprofessional education, there continues to be some uncertainty about the actual impact of this type of education. This is where systematic review work examining the effects of interprofessional education (Barr *et al.* 1999; Zwarenstein *et al.* 1999; Koppel *et al.* 2001; Cooper *et al.* 2001 and Freeth *et al.* 2002) is beginning to prove invaluable.

Ultimately, interprofessional education should have a pay-off in terms of producing effective collaboration and better quality patient care.

Evidence therefore is needed that clearly demonstrates the benefits and costs associated with interprofessional education. Such evidence will mean that this type of activity can withstand scepticism and criticism from all its potential stakeholders (e.g. policy-makers, managers, lecturers, students and clients/patients). This issue is re-visited in Chapter 7.

Implementation: pre- or post-qualification?

A national survey conducted by CAIPE in 1995 (Barr and Waterton 1996) found that work-based examples outnumbered university based by two to one and that post-qualification outnumbered pre-qualification by almost three to one. Prior to 2000 the bulk of interprofessional education therefore occurred in the post-qualification sector (Pirrie *et al.* 1998). Post-qualification programmes are also less constrained. All rather than part of the programme may be shared. The pattern of study is usually part-time enabling participants to relate theory and practice. Content has tradition-ally typically included updating knowledge, strengthening academic foun-dations, introducing new practice methods and preparing students for new roles and career progression (Storrie 1992).

An important question therefore relates to the most effective stage of introducing interprofessional education. The associated literature offers two schools of thought. Advocates of the first school (e.g. Dombeck 1997) argue that interprofessional education is better left until after qualifica-tion. By this time, it is argued, students have sufficiently developed the professional experience and confidence needed to draw upon their learn-ing with other professional groups. In contrast, advocates of the second school of thought (e.g. Tope 1996), maintain that interprofessional education is effective if delivered before qualification when students have not been socialised into their own professions and developed the negative attitudes that are often formed in this socialisation process. However, issues related to the introduction of interprofessional education are more complex than the arguments presented here suggest. The effectiveness (or not) of implementing and, more importantly, sustaining interprofes-sional education is dependent upon a range of political, organisational, educational and cultural factors.

Implementation: political, organisational, educational and cultural factors

Establishing interprofessional education is generally regarded as a problematic venture. This is due to the need for course developers to navigate their way round a number of factors: political, organisational, educational and cultural.

Political factors

The status quo is rarely identified as an option for the future (British Medical Association 2002). Yet many of the practices in health and social care are steeped in the vestiges of the last century. The considerable complexity of modernising the workforce is coupled with a backdrop of professions and organisations that often seek to defend themselves against change (Humphris and Masterson 2000). The changes and flexibilities sought from the workforce raise fundamental questions about how far reforms are willing to go in challenging the existing medical hegemony (Cameron 2000).

Organisational factors

Pirrie *et al.* (1998) have helpfully summarised various organisation considerations into 'intra-institutional' and 'extra-institutional' inhibitors. The former include: imbalances in student numbers; finding suitable accommodation for large and small group teaching; access to library and information technology facilities and timetabling problems across groups with discrete discipline-specific curricula. Often, intra-institutional inhibitors are complicated by wider extra-institutional inhibitors. These include disparate professional bodies; unsynchronised validation cycles; separate funding streams and competition between HE Institutions.

Educational factors

The introduction of interprofessional education is compounded by the existence of a number of educational factors that all need to be addressed if this type of education is to be successful.

Interprofessional education is likely to be more effective if undertaken on a recurrent basis, that is, not just a one-off in the student's learning experience. Given the historically socio-political imbalances that have existed between health and social care professions (Hugman 1991), it is also often argued that any interprofessional course demands equality between participants. The approach taken needs to recognise and acknowledge the diversity of the learning group and to ensure a positive experience for all involved. It is also recommended that this type of activity should be undertaken in professionally 'neutral' learning environments (Parsell *et al.* 1998), between equal numbers of students to ensure that one professional group does not dominate learning activities (Funnell *et al.* 1992).

Effective facilitation is a crucial requirement. Clearly facilitating interprofessional groups is a difficult task. As well as having a good knowledge of group learning theories, facilitation needs practical skills, experience and confidence to meet the differing demands of an interprofessional group. Research suggests that facilitators can be inconsistent in their work with different professional groups (Freeth and Nicol 1998; Reeves 2000). Where interprofessional education does not meet students' learning needs in terms of developing their profession specific competencies, resistance to collaborative activities can be generated (Fallsberg and Hammar 2000; Reeves and Freeth 2002). The process adopted should be interesting, relevant to the professional learning experience and practice and manageable. Finally, clear statements about learning expectations and learning outcomes provide important understandings of the process for staff and students as well as setting achievable goals.

Cultural factors

Course organisers need to be mindful of the potential impact of early professional socialisation processes. For example, a study undertaken by Pryce and Reeves (1997), found that first year medical, nursing and dental students have already developed a range of deeply embedded stereotypical notions of one another's professional groups. Such perceptions may lead students to see little value in learning together. This may also affect their motivation to learn and colour their subsequent interaction with other student groups (Barnes *et al.* 2000). Given it's relatively new and untested status, academic staff may also be sceptical of the value of interprofessional education for those involved in developing and/or delivering an interprofessional initiative. Clearly any of the above factors, singularly or collectively, will complicate the development and implementation of interprofessional education. In addition, groundbreaking projects need careful management and sensible support. Sustaining interprofessional initiatives is as challenging as initiating interprofessional developments.

Sustaining initiatives

Given its relatively new and untested status, staff may be sceptical of the value of interprofessional education. For those involved in developing and/or delivering interprofessional programmes, such reactions can seriously undermine the potential success of an interprofessional initiative. It is often recommended that only committed staff should be involved with this activity (Reeves and Freeth 2002). Without the support of these enthusiasts, interprofessional programmes are unlikely to be sustained and embedded over time (Freeth 2001).

Much of HEI's experience of developing interprofessional learning and teaching is based on a large number of small-term projects. Although some of these projects have given pointers to the potential value of interprofessional education, as 'development projects', these initiatives rarely make connections with mainstream undergraduate or postgraduate education. Short-term projects also tend to atrophy when the funding ceases. It is clear that a piecemeal approach to education commissioning will not generate a lasting commitment to interprofessional learning and teaching, as part of mainstream provision. Issues that require further discussion include:

- Revisiting the true cost of interprofessional education delivery.
- Investing in teacher staff development. Interprofessional e-learning without appropriate staff development will present challenges.
- Commissioning new pathways and routes based on future service development.
- Utilising common quality assurance mechanisms across the professions in theory and practice.
- Ensuring common and consistent student support mechanisms.
- Accepting flexible output.
- Investing in accommodation.

Conclusion

'The NHS Plan' provides HEIs with many opportunities to extend their relationship with the NHS. In particular, there is a current policy emphasis on working in partnership with the NHS to deliver post-qualification outcomes, which reflect and support service and the workforce modernisation agenda (DOH 2003a). Fitness of purpose for the next generation of health professionals is being conceptualised in policy documents in terms of shared core knowledge and competencies, team working, flexibility and potential skills transferability.

In outlining these aspirations, policy-makers contribute to the conceptual confusion between interprofessional, multiprofessional, shared and common learning, often using these terms interchangeably. Whether it is helpful to put so much emphasis upon common studies is another matter. Persuasive arguments have been put for adjusting or redressing the balance between common and specialist studies (Tope 1996). The danger lies in taking the argument to extremes, thereby detracting from the distinctive contribution that each profession makes to service delivery over emphasis upon 'common' or 'core' studies also runs counter to strongly held beliefs in interprofessional education. One might also argue that patients and clients receive the highest standards of healthcare in specialist referral centres. A policy focus on developing 'common' or 'core' studies might divert resources from developing specialist knowledge and skills learning, in the longer term, to a decline in standards of care at specialist centres but on overall improvement in standards across healthcare. Whilst the value of specialist care must not be underestimated, it may also come at a price: a lack of investment in generalist skills and the poor co-ordination of services. Finding an appropriate balance between specialist and generalist skills is a key issue facing all healthcare systems in the future (Kendall and Lissaur 2003).

There also appears to be a disconnection between policy aspirations and operational realities. However, the realisation of the government's service and modernisation agenda will require a cultural change within HEIs, service, medical deaneries, professional organisations and Workforce Development Confederations. In particular the existing medical hegemony will need to be challenged. Successful implementation of post-qualifying interprofessional education will also rest on partnership between these agencies. The concept and practice of interprofessional education also needs to be developed into a more rigorous discipline with a robust evidence-based approach that demonstrates a real impact on health status, health services and professional practice (cf. Chapter 7). Finally, interprofessional learning should not be viewed as the end, but as a means to evolve and redesign the relationship between health and social care professionals and the needs of the population.

References

Barnes, D, Carpenter, J and Dickinson, C (2000) Interprofessional Education for Community Mental Health: Attitudes to Community Care and Professional Stereotypes. *Social Work Education*, **19**(6), 565–83.

Barr, H (1996) *Perspectives on Shared Learning*. London: CAIPE.

Barr, H (2002) *Interprofessional Education Today, Yesterday and Tomorrow: A Review.* London: CAIPE.

Barr, H, Hammick, M, Koppel, I and Reeves, S (1999) Evaluating Interprofessional Education: Two Systematic Reviews for Health and Social Care. *British Educational Research Journal,* **25**(4), 533–44.

Barr, H and Waterton, S (1996) Interprofessional Educational in Health and Social Care in the United Kingdom: Report of a CAIPE Survey. London: CAIPE.

British Medical Association (2002) The Future Healthcare Workforce. HPERU Discussion Paper 9. London: BMA.

Cameron, A (2000) New Role Developments. In Developing New Clinical Roles: A Guide for Health Professionals, Humphris, D and Masterson, A (eds) London: Churchill Livingstone, 7–24.

Centre for the Advancement of Interprofessional Education (CAIPE) (1997) *Interprofessional Education – A Definition.* London: CAIPE. www.caipe.org.uk.

Cooper, H, Carlisle, C, Gibbs, T and Watkins, C (2001) Developing an Evidence Base for Interdisciplinary Learning: A Systematic Review. *Journal of Advanced Nursing,* **35**(2), 228–37.

Department of Health (1997) *The New NHS: Modern, Dependable.* London: HMSO.

Department of Health (2000a) *The NHS Plan: A Plan for Investment, a Plan for Reform.* London: HMSO.

Department of Health (2000b) A Health Service of All the Talents: Developing the NHS Workforce, Consultation Document. London: DOH.

Department of Health (2001) *Working Together – Learning Together: A Framework for Lifelong Learning for the NHS.* London: DOH.

Department of Health (2002a) *Developing a Shared Framework for Health Professional Learning Beyond Registration.* London: HMSO.

Department of Health (2002b) Unfinished Business: Proposals for Reform for the Senior House Officer Grade: A Paper for Consultation. London: DOH.

Department of Health (2003) Learning for Delivery: Making a Connection Between Post Qualification Learning and Changing Continuing Professional Development and Service Planning. DOH (draft report).

Dombeck, M (1997) Professional Personhood: Training Territoriality and Tolerance. *Journal of Interprofessional Care,* **11**, 9–21.

Fallsberg, M and Hammar, M (2000) Strategies and Focus at an Integrated Interprofessional Training Ward. *Journal of Interprofessional Care,* **14**, 337–50.

Finch, J (2000) Interprofessional Education and Teamworking: A View from the Educational Provider. *British Medical Journal,* **321**, 1138–40.

Freeth, D and Nicol, M (1998) Learning Clinical Skills: An Interprofessional Approach. *Nurse Education Today,* **18**, 455–61.

Freeth, D, Hammick, M, Koppel, I, Reeves, S and Barr, H (2002) A Critical Review of Evaluations of Interprofessional Education, Learning and Teaching Support Network Health Sciences and Practice, London: LTSN.

Funnell, P, Gill, J and Ling, J (1992) Competence Through Interprofessional Shared Learning. In D Saunders and P Pace (eds) *Developing and Measuring Competence, (Aspects of Education and Training Technology XXV)*. London: Kogan Page.

Glen, S (2001) Transdisciplinary Education: Tensions and Contradictions? *NT Research*, **6**, 807–16.

Hale, C (2002) *Questioning the Conventional Wisdom*. www.ipr.org

Horsburgh, M, Lamdin, R and Williamson, E (2001) Multiprofessional Learning: The Attitudes of Medical, Nursing and Pharmacy Students to Shared Learning. *Medical Education*, **35**, 876–83.

Hugman, R (1991) *Power in the Caring Professions*. Basingstoke: MacMillan.

Humphris, D and Macleod, Clark J (2002) *Shaping a Vision for a 'New Generation' Workforce*. Southampton: University of Southampton.

Humphris, D and Masterson, A (2000) *New Clinical Roles: A Guide for Healthcare Professions*. London: Harcourt Brace.

Jay, P (1979) (Chair) Report of the Committee of Enquiry into Mental Handicap Nursing and Care. London: HMSO.

Kendall, L and Lissaur, R (2003) *The Future Health Worker*. London: Institute of Policy, Practice and Research.

Kennedy *et al.* (2001) Bristol Royal Infirmary Inquiry, Final Report. London: DOH.

Koppel, I, Barr, H, Reeves, S, Freeth, D and Hammick, M (2001) Establishing a Systematic Approach to Evaluating the Effectiveness of Interprofessional Education. *Issues in Interdisciplinary Care*, **3**(1), 41–50.

Miller, C, Ross, N and Freeman, M (1999) *Shared Learning and Clinical Teamwork: New Directions in Education for Multiprofessional Practice*. London: ENB.

NHS South West Regional Office (2002) Learning and Working Together, NHS South West.

NHSE (1999) *Agenda for Change: Modernising the NHS Pay System*. London: HMSO.

Parsell, G, Spalding, R and Bligh, J (1998) *Shared Goals, Shared Learning: Evaluation of a Multiprofessional Course for Undergraduate Students*. Medical Education, **32**, 304–11.

Pirrie, A, Elsegood, J and Hall, J (1998) Evaluating Multidisciplinary Education in Health Care. Final Report of a 24 Month Funded Study. London: DOH.

Pryce, A and Reeves, S (1997) An Exploratory Research Project of a Multidisciplinary Education Module for Medical, Dental and Nursing Students. City University Internal Research Report, ISBN 1900804 06 9.

Reeves, S (2000) Community-based Interprofessional Education for Medical, Nursing and Dental Students. *Health and Social Care in the Community*, **8**, 269–76.

Reeves, S and Freeth, D (2002) The London Training Ward: An Innovative Interprofessional Learning Initiative. *Journal of Interprofessional Care*, **16**, 41–52.

Storrie, J (1992) Mastering Interprofessionalism – An Enquiry into the Development of Masters Programmes with an Interprofessional Focus. *Journal of Interprofessional Care*, **6**(3), 253–9.

Tope, R (1996) *Integrated Interdisciplinary Learning Between the Health and Social Care Professions: A Feasibility Study*. Aldershot: Avebury.

Zwarenstein, M, Atkins, J, Barr, H, Hammick, M, Koppel, I and Reeves, S (1999) A Systematic Review of Interprofessional Education. *Journal of Interprofessional Care*, **13**(4) 417–24.

Web addresses

Centre for the Advancement of Interprofessional Education: www.caipe.org.uk.

Centre for Health Sciences and Practice: www.health/ltsn.ac.uk.

University of Southampton: The New Generation Project: http://www.mhbs.soton.ac.uk/newgeneration/about.htm.

Healthwork UK (2001) National Occupational Standards: www.healthwork.co.uk/standards.htm.

Healthwork UK (2001) Ordering National Occupational Standards: www.healthwork.co.uk/qualifications/order.htm.

2

User and Carer Involvement in Interprofessional Post-qualifying Education and Training

Tony Leiba

Introduction

This chapter aspires to raise some issues, which are relevant to user and carer involvement in the education and training of health and social care professionals. It is a plea for users and carers to move from being absent from education and training development and delivery, to being active participants in such activities.

There is a belief that more user and carer collaboration and participation is a good thing. Furthermore, there is evidence of extensive user and carer participation in the delivery of mental health care through the processes of the Care Planning Approach (Anthony and Crawford, 2000). Users have increasingly expressed that they are no longer prepared to be passive and are engaging in meaningful challenges to traditional structures and processes in health and social services (Rogers and Pilgrim, 1991). User and carer groups are becoming more organised, articulate and informed, and questioning the health and social care system that has set itself up as 'we know best' and should not be questioned. Those responsible for the education and training of professionals have increased the opportunities for students from different professions to learn together. However, it is still relatively rare for service users or carers to contribute to interprofessional education (Tope, 1998). More recently Hanson and Mitchell (2001) argue that there is much rhetorical support for user involvement in nurse education. However, active involvement cannot develop without recognition of the need by educators, and the provision of appropriate preparation for users and carers. Furthermore, Forrest *et al.* (2000) argues that there is some promising research demonstrating that user involvement is taking place in the work of Wood and Wilson-Barnett (1999). However, Forrest *et al.* (2000) adds that this must be built upon over time to involve every aspect of curriculum development and avoid tokenism.

Indeed, despite the rhetoric of partnership, collaboration and the growth of consumerism, users' and carers' views and contributions are often undervalued. The concerns here will be to examine the involvement of users and carers in the planning and delivery of post-qualifying education and training in mental health services.

Background

The value of involving users in the education and training of mental health and social care workers has been emphasised in a number of reports: Pulling Together (Sainsbury Centre for Mental Health, 1997), Users' Voices (Rose, D, 2000), The NHS Plan (Department of Health, 2000), The National Service Framework for Mental Health (Department of Health, 1999); and Users' Views on Training for Community Care (Department of Health, Social Services Inspectorate, 1994).

The development of user and carer involvement has gone hand in hand with the consumerism and partnership principle, which promotes collaborative working between users and carers and service providers. Furthermore, the shift from a service-led culture to one which is needs-led, should provide for a more user sensitive mental health and social care service delivery.

The notion of collaboration in education and training has been firmly placed on the agenda for change and it is a clear challenge to professionals who have always dictated what is to happen to users. Users and carers collaboration in education and training should be sought for the development of teaching methods and course content. Such a collaboration would make available: the users experiences of mental disorder; their carers experiences; enhance the students' understanding of the social context of peoples' problems, service users definition of what they need and what experiences they have had of the services; the enabling of educationalists and students to begin to appreciate the individual experience of mental distress; and to provide a way forward for the promotion of user sensitive care.

Shields (1985) argued that by seeking users' and carers' participation it may be possible to challenge professionals who traditionally have dictated what is to happen to users. Also that in a democracy the professionals are accountable to the public, and that a way in which this accountability can be achieved is through user and carer participation. According to Edwards (2000) the 1990s saw mental health service users and their carers finding their voice, a voice that is increasingly demanding to be listened to. The attention now being paid to eliciting users' and carers' views, indicate a paradigm shift, from considering users as objects of care and treatments to users being participants in their own care and treatments.

This cultural shift in the provision of mental health services is needed if staff are to work interprofessionally and collaborate with users and carers to provide user centred care (Department of Health, Social Services Inspectorate, 1994; Sainsbury Centre, 1997). These requirements imply that post-qualifying professional education and training should be interprofessional and that there is an important role for service users and carers in its provision (Lindow and Morris, 1995). The Sainsbury Centre (1997) stressed that in order to create an effective mental health workforce, active dialogue must take place between the professions, employers and a wide range of stakeholders, particularly including users and carers. However, service users and carers have reported that many professionals are reluctant to listen to them, and too often, interpret their opinions as a challenge to professional expertise (Towns *et al.*, 1997). The consumerist approach (Department of Health, 1989), regarded service users as consumers of a care market and able to exercise choice in the services they used. Barnes *et al.* (2000) argued that the care market was at best a quasi-market in which service users had little or no choice, were not in control of the funds with which to wield consumer power and that consultation often took place after decisions had been made and so limiting the influence of service users.

Indeed, despite the rhetoric of partnership and the growth of consumerism, users and carers views and contributions are often undervalued. Developments in consumerism and user involvement have been influenced by critical commentaries made by users of existing service provisions. Bury (1997) argues that consumerism has involved major changes in organisation and outlook in the National Health Service by moving the focus away from the providers or producer of health and social care to users as customers. Annandale (1996) in a study of nurse' and midwives' views of risk, found that they perceived consumerism as putting a greater emphasis on patients rights, resulting in a lack of trust between practitioner and patient, more informal complaints, more formal complaints and litigation. Concluding that authority has shifted from the provider to the consumer and that practitioners have lost their confidence in their autonomy to practice.

Users as consumers are demanding that providers have sensitive regards for diversity in providing for their needs. DOH (1991) outlines ten rights and nine national standards. However, users as consumers of health and social care cannot choose their care. This puts the whole ethics of what providers offer to users in question. Users' rights under the Patients Charter is mediated by, general practitioners, fundholders and purchaser health trusts who choose what services to provide. Furthermore, health and social care needs are difficult to specify and any agreement for services often have to be flexible enough to allow for variation of interpretation. Service users and carers as consumers can assist health and social care professionals in how they address and provide for their diversity of needs, through being a part of the educational and training processes such professionals receive.

According to Wood and Wilson-Barnett (1999) listening to users being critical or angry about professional practice can be uncomfortable and can lead to professionals becoming defensive. Staff may feel reluctant to let go of the security felt by their professional status, arguing that those in distressed states are unsuitable for collaborative relationships. Furthermore, being constantly confronted by the distressing aspects of mental distress can result in staff distancing themselves, making it difficult for users and professionals to regard themselves as partners. Such a situation is compounded by what Hopton (1994) refers to as a culture in which the mental health user is thought of as an inferior person. However, Wood and Wilson-Barnett (1999) found that students exposed to user involvement in the classroom were less likely than others to use jargon and to be more able to empathise with users' experiences of distress.

The involvement of users in education and training is likely to increase their self-esteem and self-confidence through being in the role of helper rather than helped (Barnes and Bowl, 2001). Therefore, helping users of mental health services to develop a positive educator trainer role may serve to diminish the sick role and at the same time enable students to recognise the value of users' personal knowledge. However, active involvement cannot develop without appropriate preparation. Users and carers will need to be prepared to work as trainers, speakers and workshop facilitators. An example of such a preparatory course for users and carers is the 'Training for growth' project at Nottingham University (Hanson and Mitchell, 2001).

Users' and carers' involvement in education and training

Simpson (1999) involved users and carers in an investigation to identify the training needs of Community Mental Health Nurses. Users and carers were asked in interviews and focused groups to consider and offer their views on the following: the skills they most valued in a Community Mental Health Nurse; care and treatments they would like Community Mental Health Nurses to do; specific issues that they would like Community Mental Health Nurses to be trained in; the involvement of carers; and the involvement of users and carers and their organisations in the education and training of Community Mental Health Nurses.

The users identified the following aspects which requires attention in the training programmes for Community Mental Health Nurses: CMHNs able to provide advice and information on medication, physical and medical problems, local services, accommodation, finances and employment; how to involve users and their carers in the care processes and in education and training initiatives; CMHNs to involve carers in care planning, to understand their important role and to help them access support networks; users wanted the training to provide CMHNs with greater awareness of the role played by carers and an understanding of their specific difficulties; CMHNs who are able to communicate jargon free whilst being aware of implicit values and attitudes; to have extensive knowledge of the local mental health services available, in particular user self-help groups; to be able to monitor mental health problems and help users deal with difficult times; and to enable CMHNs to demonstrate greater inclusion of the viewpoints and experiences of users and carers in mental health nurse education.

Issues around medication management were repeatedly mentioned. Users wanted CMHNs to have a wide knowledge of medications, their side effects and contraindications and to spend more time listening and talking to them about medicines. There is evidence form the work of

Dubyan and Quinn (1996) that a closer working relationship and effective medication management can result in user satisfaction, compliance and successful self-management.

Despite all the documentations which states that users' and carers' involvement are central to the Care programme Approach (Department of Health, 1990), Simpson (1999) suggests that CMHNs still fail to involve users and carers fully when developing care plans. This results in users claiming that the Care Programme Approach, Keyworker and multiagency working remains either as not happening, or not being seen to happen.

Users and their organisations want CMHNs to demonstrate more awareness of the role played by the voluntary services and of the mistrust, suspicion and even disrespect that may exist between the statutory and the voluntary services. Users want to see rights and empowerment made central to CMHNs education and training. Users also felt that more training was needed to address the issues of discrimination, oppression and stigma, so equipping the CMHN with the necessary skills to help the range of people who face prejudice within the mental health service, including, women, ethnic groups, gay people and the homeless.

The carers identified training needs of CMHNs, which were similar to those of the user group. They pointed out that the user's family and carer had been overlooked in nurse training and that carers would welcome involvement in all levels of nurse education and training.

Barnes *et al.* (2000) evaluated a post-qualifying programme of interprofessional education in community mental health. Service users were involved in the development and delivery of a course. The course was for staff from health, social services and voluntary organisations working in community mental health. The curriculum development membership included representatives from all the stakeholders including users as full members. It was recognised that preparation of the users was necessary if they are to feel comfortable and participate fully. The focus of the course was to address user concerns and some examples of user defined outcomes were: staff should treat service users with respect, not as labels; professionals should have knowledge about services, including advocacy and user groups; staff should be able to provide information about how to complain; staff should know how to involve users in the assessment of their needs; staff from different agencies and different professions should learn to work together; staff should know how to involve service users, carers and their families in developing care plans; staff should be able to provide information about legislation and user's rights; the different knowledge and perspectives of professionals should be valued; and staff should be able to provide information about medication.

Some of the participants felt that the users contributions had been too antagonistic while others appreciated the way in which users presenters had spoken about their own experiences of receiving multidisciplinary mental health care. Participants described initiatives in their workplaces aimed at making users the central focus of their mental health services. Participants were also made aware of the disempowering aspects of the psychiatric system and the limitations of the medical model (Barnes *et al.*, 2000).

The investigation by Turner *et al.* (2000) 'Listening to and learning from the family carer's story: an innovative approach in interprofessional education' provides an example of carer involvement in interprofessional education around palliative care. Although this was not strictly a mental health focused initiative, there are important education and training issues which can be transferred to the mental health setting. The investigators at the outset were concerned about the carers, preparation for the workshops, because they only received a short telephone call asking them to participate, followed by information on date, time and venue and that they would be asked about their experiences of caring for their relative. The investigators were also influenced by the idea that health care education may be more effective if it is set within a real life context and not only taught theoretically. Schon (1987) articulated the inadequacy of theory to prepare practitioners for the complex and problematic world of practice, and the challenges of matching what is learned in the classroom to real life clinical situations. In the workshop the interprofessional participants from nursing, medicine, social work, occupational therapy and physiotherapy elicited the carers' experience of caring for someone who is terminally ill. The exact workshop tasks were: to hear the carer's story; which different professionals were involved; how was their input co-ordinated; who was the key person who made or didn't make it work; and what would have made the care provided better for the patient, carer and the professionals.

Talking to carers allowed the participants to gain insights into their own profession and health care in general. They were made aware of the lack of knowledge carers had about the body, disease, treatment, prognosis systems of care, the interface between health and social services, policy and funding. This led them to see the importance of communication, not taking anything for granted and that a chance action or statement on the part of a professional might have a lasting impact for good or ill. They learned about how care was seen through the eyes of the carers', that care needs may change rapidly and that services are not always flexible enough to meet these needs. They felt that they learned about real situations, the inadequacies of the system as well as the things that worked well.

The carers were positive about the workshops and its contribution to the teaching. However, they considered their preparation to be inadequate and they felt they did not know what they were coming to and wanted more specific information. They welcomed the opportunity to unload and to present the real situations they were in to the participants.

This initiative resulted in students gaining valuable insights into the carers' knowledge and learned about the actual situations rather than textbook ones.

User involvement in research

The role of evidence is seen as being at the heart of effective planning and delivery of health and social care. In providing education and training research activities must take place and involve users and health and social care professionals in collaboration. Truman and Raine (2001) argues that participatory evaluative research involving users, is necessary in the creation of an evidence-based health care provision within a community mental health service. Furthermore, that users who participate in the research process in a meaningful way facilitate changes in the way that research is commissioned and assessed so that the nature of user involvement may become viable. User involvement in mental health research is essential if service provision is to be responsive to their needs (Hickey and Kipping, 1998).

Chamberlain and Rogers (1990) sees user involvement as a right, with the service user being best placed to advise, shape and develop services. Participatory research therefore, provides a means of shifting the balance of knowledge production back in the direction of vulnerable groups, providing those who take part in it with a greater sense of ownership over the findings, and at the same time alerting the powerful research commissioning bodies such as the Department of Health that models of research must be used that insist on the involvement of users from the onset.

Furthermore, the bodies which are responsible for the Research Assessment Exercise in Universities, along with other funding bodies such as the Kings Fund, now require uses and carers to be involved in the commissioning, evaluation and assessment of research related to health and social care. In 1997 the Mental Health Foundation published 'Knowing Our Own Minds' a report based on a survey conducted with mental health service users. The whole project was led, steered, researched and written by people who identified themselves as users or survivors of mental health services. Today, in much health and social care provision, involving users and carers in monitoring and evaluation exercises is now a requirement. Current examples of these processes are evident in the monitoring of the standards of the National Service Framework for Mental Health and the Commission for Health Improvement.

Users and carers being involved in the research process may not necessarily mean equal empowerment, because although users were being involved in research, they remained the subjects of that research in an unequal relationship where the power to interpret and to know remains in the hands of the researcher. User and carer involvement in research challenges the traditional approach where they are the subjects of the research to having a say in how the research is conducted and to be a full part of the collection of information, the analysis and the writing of the report. The 'Do It Yourself Guide to Survivor Research' (Mental Health Foundation, 1999) and The 'Strategies for Living Research Report' (Mental Health Foundation, 2000) takes the reader through the processes and training needed to do effective user and carer involvement research.

Fenge (2002) arguing from a social work perspective suggests that participatory research can be used to encourage older people, and older people from ethnic minority groups such as ethnic and gay elders to have a voice in defining their needs and experiences. Within social work practice anti-discriminatory practice is a dominant theme, and when working with older people anti-ageism practice is central. Therefore, collaborative research between older users and social workers could increase the knowledge and understanding about the needs and experiences of this group and the great diversity within them. Such collaborative research should benefit users, when social work educationalists using the research findings, ensure that tomorrow's practitioners have new insights into the needs of older people and older minorities.

The implications of user and carer led research for the future service provision, health and social care research and for education and training are manifold. It is through such research that a clearer picture will emerge of what constitutes good practice in mental health treatment and care, and getting such information translated into the education and training of health and social care professionals. For mental health and social care professionals who are under the impression that user led research will only produce a litany of negative findings, the 'Strategies for Living Report' (Mental Health Foundation, 2000), demonstrates that users are quick to praise mental health services they see as examples of good practice. It is through such examples of good practice, revealed by user led research that mental health services can benefit.

Facilitating user involvement in education and training

Providing health and social care in the mental health services, could be conceived as giving people a greater individual say in how they live their lives and the services they need to help them to do so. In order to achieve this user and carer involvement is essential. Such an involvement must not remain embedded in rhetoric but have the same importance as collaboration and interprofessional working is between the professionals. Much to date is written about interprofessional education and training between professionals and considerably less on the involvement of users and carers in such initiatives. There has been an increase in the opportunities for the different professionals in health and social care to work together, in the hope that this will promote improved collaboration in practice (Parsell *et al.*, 1998).

To start to address this involvement in education and training there must be strong backing from senior agency managers, senior education managers and practical and moral support from operational staff and lecturers. Other important considerations must include: users and carers being involved from the start on a equal basis, and the plans must reflect their concerns as well as those of the professionals; there must be enough time to build trust between service users and the professionals; working over time planning and developing an educational initiative is a good way for developing trust and an equal relationship; and users and carers need time and money to develop their networks, ideas and to operationalise them. When holding meetings and training events, attention to practical details is essential for example, accessible venues, public transport, availability of parking, times of events planned to enable participants to function in their domestic life, the provision of help with substitute carers, the provision of interpreters as is required. It must be remembered that service users and carers often feel anxious about getting involved. Meetings and training events is unfamiliar to most people, users and carers are likely to feel anxious, unconfident and at a disadvantage in the face of confident professionals. Professionals may also feel anxious about engaging with users and carers. They may fear criticism or that they will not be able to meet demands. Involving users and carers means challenging and changing traditional attitudes and ways of working, and it is difficult for staff to participate in the reappraisal of their jobs.

In order to provide interprofessional education and training between users, carers and health and social care professionals, there is a need to have effective facilitation of such events. Educational facilitation according to Burrows (1997, p. 401) is, 'A goal-oriented dynamic process in which participants work together in an atmosphere of genuine mutual respect, in order to learn through critical reflection.' The facilitator must create an atmosphere conducive to participation so that the participants can be questioning, probing, challenging, encouraging critical reflection to create a greater awareness in the individual of his or her beliefs, values and assumptions. The facilitator must ensure that he or she add to the potential for learning within the group without taking away from participants the control of their own learning. A suggested plan of facilitation could be: the initiation of group involvement and begin to create a climate of collaborative learning; establishing negotiated ground rules which include confidentiality and freedom of expression; and the development of trust, safety, respect, non-judgemental attitudes, honesty, active listening and participation.

A most crucial aspect of facilitation is the intervening in the group process in the right way at the right time when there is conflict or confusion, remembering that learning takes place when we move from conflict and or confusion to clarity.

Conclusion

If education and training programmes are to prepare professionals for the world of practice, they need to draw on real life situations which gives health and social care professionals an opportunity to meet and talk to users and carers. Work needs to be done to evaluate long-term outcomes such as, understanding the users and carers perspectives and expectations, change in attitudes, improved communications and that such an interprofessional teaching and learning exposure leads to improved care for users.

References

Annandale, E (1996) Working on the Front Line: Risk, Culture and Nursing in the New NHS. *The Sociological Review*, **44**(3), 416–51.

Anthony, P and Crawford, P (2000) Service User Involvement in Care Planning: The Mental Health Nurse's Perspective. *Journal of Psychiatric and Mental Health Nursing*, **7**, 425–34.

Barnes, D, Carpenter, J and Bailey, D (2000) Partnerships with Service Users in Interprofessional Education for Community Mental Health: A Case Study. *Journal of Interprofessional Care*, **14**(2), 189–200.

Barnes, M and Bowl, R (2001) Involving Service Users in Training. *The Journal of Practice and Development*, **7**(2), 5–11.

Bury, M (1997) *Health and Illness in a Changing Society*. London; Routledge.

Burrows, D E (1997) Facilitation: A Concept Analysis. *Journal of Advanced Nursing*, **25**, 396–404.

Chamberlain, J and Rogers, J A (1990) Planning a Community Based Mental Health System: Perspectives of Service Recipients. *American Psychologist*, **45**(11), 1241–44.

Department of Health (1989) *Caring for people*, Cm 849. London: HMSO.

Department of Health (1990) *The Care Programme Approach for People with Mental Illness* [HC (90) 23]. London: HMSO.

Department of Health (1991) *Patients Charter*. London: HMSO.

Department of Health, Social Services Inspectorate (1994) *Users' Views on Training for Community Care*. London, Department of Health, Social Services Inspectorate.

Department of Health (1999) *The National Framework for Mental Health*. London: HMSO.

Department of Health (2000) *The NHS Plan. A Plan for Investment. A Plan for Reform*. London: The Stationary Office.

Dubyan, J and Quinn, C (1996) The Self-management of Psychiatric Medications: A Pilot Study. *Journal of Psychiatric and Mental Health Nursing*, **3**, 297–302.

Edwards, K (2000) Service Users and Mental Health Nursing. *Journal of Psychiatric and Mental Health Nursing*, **7**, 555–65.

Fenge, A L (2002) Practising Partnership-Participatory Inquiry with Older People. *Social Work Education*, **21**(2), 172–81.

Forrest, S, Risk, I, Masters, H and Brown, N (2000) Mental Health Service Users Involvement in Nurse Education: Exploring the Issues. *Journal of Psychiatric and Mental Health Nursing*, **7**, 51–7.

Hanson, B and Mitchell, D (2001) Involving Mental Health Service Users in the Classroom: A Course of Preparation. *Nurse Education in Practice*, **1**, 120–6.

Hickey, G and Kipping, C (1998) Exploring the Concept of User Involvement in Mental Health Through a Participation Continuum. *Journal of Clinical Nursing*, **7**, 83–8.

Hopton, J (1994) User Involvement in the Education of Mental Health Nurses. An Evaluation of Possibilities. *Critical Social Policy*, **42**, 47–60.

Lindow, V and Morris, J (1995) *Service Users Involvement. Synthesis of Findings and Experience in the Field of Community Care*. York: Joseph Roundtree Foundation.

Mental Health Foundation (1999) *DIY Guide to Survivor Research*. London: Mental Health Foundation.

Mental Health Foundation (2000) *Strategies for Living Research Report*. London: Mental Health Foundation.

Parsell, G, Spalding, R and Bligh, J (1998) Shared Goals, Shared Learning: Evaluation of a Multiprofessional Course for Undergraduate Students. *Medical Education*, **32**, 304–11.

Rogers, A and Pilgrim, D (1991) Pulling Down Churches – Accounting for the British Mental Health Users' Movement. *Sociology of Health and Illness*, **13**, 129–48.

User's Voices (Rose 2000) London: Sainsbury Centre Publication.

Sainsbury Centre for Mental Health (1997) *Pulling Together*. London: Sainsbury Centre Publication.

Schon, D (1987) *Educating the Reflective Practitioner*. San Francisco: Jossey Bass.

Shields, P (1985) The Consumer View of Psychiatry. *Hospital and Health Services Review*, May, 117–19.

Simpson, A (1999) Creating Alliances: The Views of Users and Carers on the Education and Training needs of Community Mental Health Nurses. *Journal of Psychiatric and Mental Health Nursing*, **6**, 347–50.

Tope, R (1998) Meeting the Challenge: Introducing Service Users and Carers into the Education Equation. *CAPIE Bulletin*, **15**, 11.

Towns, N, Foster, R, Grant, S, Crosby, D, Emmerson, P, Williams, M, Edington, C and Mountain, L (1997) The County Durham Service Users and Carers Forum. *Journal of interprofessional Care*, **ii**, 139–47.

Truman, C and Raine, P (2001) Involving Users in Evaluation: The Social Relations of User Participation in Health Research. *Critical Public Health*, **11**(3), 216–29.

Turner, P, Sheldon, F, Coles, C, Mountford, B, Hillier, R, Radway, P and Wee, B (2000) Listening to and Learning from the Family Carer's Story: An Innovative Approach in Interprofessional Education. *Journal of Interprofessional Care*, **14**(4), 388–95.

Wood, J and Wilson-Barnett, J (1999) The Influence of User Involvement on the Learning of Mental Health Nursing Students. *NTResearch*, **4**(4), 257–72.

3

Work-based Interprofessional Education for Community Mental Health Teams

Scott Reeves

Introduction

This chapter describes a pilot project that offered a series of interprofessional workshops to two community mental health teams (CMHTs) based in London. These workshops provided both CMHTs with an opportunity to participate in a team-based learning experience that aimed at enhancing their knowledge and understanding of interprofessional collaboration. The chapter presents details on the development, delivery and evaluation of these workshops. Findings from the evaluation are presented and discussed before conclusions are drawn.

Background literature

For over 20 years, national policy has called for better collaboration between mental health care practitioners (e.g. Department of Health and Social Security, 1980, Department of Health, 1996, 1997, 1998). However, it appears that these policy recommendations have not comprehensively taken root at practice level. Research into the practice of mental health staff continues to indicate that their collaborative work is inhibited by a number of factors. These include uncertainties around overlapping professional roles within mental health teams (Sainsbury Health Centre, 1997), confusion over clear management lines of different mental health staff (Øvretveit, 1993) and a growing tension around the introduction of generic working within mental health teams (Brown *et al.*, 2000).

Interprofessional education is commonly suggested as a possible route to resolving some of the problems undermining effective collaboration (National Health Service Executive, 1996; Department of Health, 2000). Within this documentation there is a shared belief that this form of education can develop the necessary attitudes, knowledge and skills to promote effective interprofessional collaboration that ultimately enhances client care.

Research into the impact of interprofessional education is beginning to demonstrate that it can help promote improved collaborative practice (e.g. Chapter 7). For example, a number of studies have found that interprofessional education can:

- Enhance understanding of different professional roles (Cook *et al.*, 1995; Long, 1996; Stein and Brown, 1995);
- Increase knowledge of teamwork (Rutter and Hagart, 1990; Donat *et al.*, 1991; Reeves, 2000);
- Improve collaborative practice (Hunter and Love, 1996; Stevens *et al.*, 1997);
- Enhance the quality of care delivered to patients (Falconer *et al.*, 1993; Brown, 2000).

To understand the impact of this form of education in a more rigorous way, systematic review work is now underway. Initial findings from a review by Koppel *et al.* (2001) suggest that this form of education can make a positive impact on collaborative practice and patient outcomes across a number of health and social care settings. These findings are supported by another review undertaken by Reeves (2001) that assessed the impact of interprofessional education specifically in mental health settings. Results from this work reveal that interprofessional education can provide positive learning experiences to mental health practitioners, strengthen understanding of collaboration and improve co-ordination of mental health teams.

Despite the encouraging evidence, both reviews have found that a large number of studies of interprofessional education tend to be of poor quality. Most research in this area tends to employ simplistic evaluative designs with little effort undertaken to understand the longer-term impact of this form of education (e.g. Chapter 7).

Project development

The initial idea for developing the workshops originated from a shared enthusiasm of interprofessional education. This enthusiasm led educationalists and practitioners to form a project steering group to develop a series of pilot interprofessional workshops for mental health staff.

Drawing upon local contacts, steering group members approached the managers of two local CMHTs ('North Team' and 'South Team'). Both were interested in participating in the project as both felt the workshops would provide their teams with useful staff development.

Working with the team managers, the steering group developed a series of three pilot interprofessional workshops. The aim of the workshops was to offer CMHT members an opportunity to discuss a range of issues relating to their interprofessional work and provide them with time to reflect upon their experience of collaboration within their team. In meeting these aims, the workshops had two main learning outcomes:

- To improve knowledge of differing professional roles and the contribution to care that each profession makes;
- To enhance understanding of working together in a collaborative manner.

It was anticipated that if this project was successful, these workshops could be delivered to larger number of CMHTs.

Delivering the workshops

Following the planning process, three weekly sessions were offered to both CMHTs. Team managers were asked to invite all the members of their respective teams to the workshops.

Each workshop lasted for around two hours and involved a number of group-based activities (see Box 3.1). All workshops were facilitated by a steering group member: an experienced mental health nurse with an extensive knowledge of interprofessional issues and expertise in facilitating interprofessional groups.

To help prepare participants, information packs containing details of the workshops and a list of suggested reading were sent to each of the

---

Workshop 1

- Small group discussions of the different professional roles/functions of each team member.
- Small group discussions of the different 'models' of team-work used by each CMHT.
- Feedback and plenary discussion.

Workshop 2

- Team discussion around a number of published papers on the subject of teamwork.
- Small group discussion of practice areas where the teams felt they were working well together and areas where it was felt they needed development.
- Feedback and plenary discussion.

Workshop 3

- Group work developing team 'action plans' (each team outlined their future intentions on developing more effective collaborative practice).
- Feedback and plenary discussion.

Box 3.1   Content of the workshops

managers for distribution among their CMHTs. To ensure that participants were clear about each of the workshops, the facilitator negotiated and agreed the content of all sessions before beginning work with the teams.

Due to heavy workloads, both managers considered it was more efficient to deliver the workshops at each team's own base, in place of their regular business meeting. However, difficulties securing space at the South Team base meant that their workshops were held at a nearby educational institution.

Evaluation – methodological approach

A formative evaluation of the workshops was undertaken to assess their impact on the two CMHTs. It was anticipated that if the workshops were considered successful, this format could be offered to larger numbers of CMHTs.

In order to obtain the range of views, perspectives and experiences connected with this educational event, a multi-method research design was employed. Previous experience of evaluating interprofessional education (e.g. Reeves and Freeth, 2002) has proved that this type of approach is advantageous in capturing the complex range of views and perspectives involved in this form of education.

The author was invited to steering group meetings. Although, the primary aim of attending these meetings was to assist with the planning of the evaluation, the author's knowledge of interprofessional education meant that he contributed, to some extent, in the development of the workshops.

Data collection

Three methods of data collection were employed: questionnaires, observations and interviews. To understand the impact of the workshops, specifically whether attitudes, perceptions, knowledge and behaviour had altered as a result of this educational event, data were collected before, during and after the initiative.

Questionnaires

To examine changes in attitudes, perceptions and knowledge resulting from the workshops, questionnaire data were collected before and after the workshops. Questionnaires were divided into five sections. The first collected biographical information. The second section collected views of interprofessional teamwork. The third collected attitudes to interprofessional education and the fourth collected views of team roles. Participants gauged their responses to questions in these sections on a six-point Likert type scale. The final section allowed participants to provide detailed responses about their expectations and experiences of the workshops.

Observations

To capture group interaction during the workshops, observations of all sessions were undertaken. Unlike the more active stance taken during steering group meetings, the author's role in this part of the project was that of a marginal participant (Hammersley and Atkinson, 1995). After outlining the purpose of the evaluation to participants at the start of the first session, the author observed each session without any further contribution.

Follow-up interviews

To examine the longer-term impact of the workshops upon participants' practice, semi-structured interviews were undertaken with both teams three months after the workshops. These data were collected by a combination of group interviews and individual telephone interviews. The latter method was employed to follow-up non-attendance at the group interviews.

Data analysis

A three-stage approach to the data analysis was undertaken. Initially, quantitative data gathered from the questionnaires were summarised. Due to the small sample size in this evaluation, tests of statistical significance were not undertaken. Secondly, qualitative data gathered from the observations and interviews were analysed thematically to explore emergent themes. Finally, triangulation of the three data sets (questionnaires, observations and interviews) was undertaken to verify and crosscheck initial findings from the first and second stage analysis.

Findings – participating teams

Two London-based CMHTs participated in this project. The first (North Team) consisted of twenty-two members, including: three administrative staff; seven community psychiatric nurses (CPNs); two psychiatrists; one occupational therapist and nine social workers (including the team manager). This team had been established as a CMHT for around four years. Their client mix centred on people with severe and enduring mental illness.

The second CMHT (South Team) comprised of nineteen members, including: two administrative staff; five CPNs (including the team manager); one psychiatrist; one psychologist two support worker; one occupational therapist; and seven social workers. In contrast, this team had only been operating as a CMHT since January 2001. This team's client mix also centred on people with severe and enduring mental illness.

Profession	North Team	South Team
Medicine	2	–
Nursing	7	5
Social worker	9	6
Occupational therapy	1	1
Support staff	–	1
Psychology	–	–
Total	19	13

Box 3.2 Workshop participation

Attendance

In total, 32 people participated in the workshops (19 from North Team and 13 from South Team). Professional representation came from social work, nursing, medicine, occupational therapy and support staff. In addition, both team managers attended the workshops (see Box 3.2).

Pre-workshop perspective

Views and attitudes

Twenty-nine participants completed a pre-workshop questionnaire. In terms of participants' views of how well their teams collaborated, the data revealed that although most participants reported that there was a co-operative atmosphere within their teams (n = 26/29), their views on issues such as team equity, professional difference and team conflict resolution were more mixed. For example, around half the participants (n = 16/29) felt that interprofessional conflict was effectively resolved in their teams, whereas others (n = 8/29) felt that conflict tended to be unresolved.

In relation to participants' role clarity, while most (n = 23/29) stated that they were confident about their individual role in the team, many were uncertain about the amount of authority they had in the team (n = 11/29) and were also unclear about the objectives for their role in the team (n = 11/29).

In contrast, participants held very favourable attitudes towards interprofessional education. For example, the vast majority of participants felt that interprofessional education could promote effective team collaboration (n = 28); could improve understanding of one another's roles (n = 28); and could be a useful tool in team building (n = 27).

Expectations

Participants were generally looking forward to the prospect of the workshops. Most felt that these sessions had potential for enhancing their understanding of the range of different professional roles that made up their CMHT. As one participant noted:

> The workshops will help us understand each others' roles better. (psychiatrist)

It was also felt that the workshops could enhance the quality of their collective work as a CMHT:

> It will provide a clearer definition of team working and collaboration which should improve our communication. (CPN)

However, for a few participants, there was a fear that attending these sessions would add increased pressure of their already heavy workloads:

> These workshops take time away from me when I have lots of things to do on my caseload. (social worker)

For some of the participants in South Team, who had to travel to the workshops, the potential problem of pressurised time was felt more acutely.

During the workshops

Observational data collected during the workshops revealed that all sessions were undertaken in a relaxed atmosphere with good interaction between participants and a positive rapport between participants and facilitator.

Workshop 1

This workshop centred upon two team activities. The first activity aimed at clarifying the different roles and functions that existed in each CMHT, the second focused on discussing the different approaches team members took with their collaborative work. It was interesting to note that during these activities, many participants raised the issue of poor attendance from their medical colleagues. This tended to result in some discussion of the difficulties collaborating with these staff. There was a shared view that medical staff, especially the senior staff, tended to work separately from the other team members.

Workshop 2

The first part of this workshop was focused on exploring participants' views of the papers they had read from the suggested reading contained in their information packs. For this activity, the facilitator spent time linking participants' experiences of collaboration with the conceptual and empirical material in these papers. Despite informing all participants (in the first workshop) of this activity, many participants had not found the time to undertake the suggested reading. Consequently, the depth of team discussions was limited to a superficial level.

The second part of the session focused on small group discussions of areas in which participants felt their teams were working effectively and areas where they felt development was needed. For South Team (where there was no medical participation) this led to another team discussion on the lack of involvement of their medical colleagues in the workshops.

Workshop 3

The final workshop focused around developing a series of interprofessional action plans. Participants worked together to plan a range of ideas that could strengthen their future collaborative practice (see Box 3.3).

Each of these action plans was then discussed and a time scale was agreed when each of these plans would be implemented within the team.

Aim: improve collaborative assessment
Co-ordinating member: CPN
Implementation: brainstorming, problem-solving, literature searching pilot study with 2–3 cases where one team member shadows another
Evaluation: pre/post data, focus on effectiveness, difficulties, user-friendliness
Time scale: 5 months

Box 3.3 An example of team action plan

Post-workshop perspective

Views and attitudes

Twenty-three participants completed a post-workshop questionnaire. These data revealed that participants' views on collaboration in their teams remained largely unaltered from the views they expressed in their pre-workshop questionnaires.

Similarly, it was found that participants' attitudes of interprofessional education also remained unchanged. Like their pre-workshop attitudes, the majority of participants maintained their favourable attitudes of interprofessional education.

However, some small improvements were made with participants' clarity of their individual roles within their teams. It was found that a slightly higher proportion felt they were certain of the amount of authority they had in the team (n = 11/23) and were also clear about the objectives for their role in the team (n = 11/23).

Workshop experiences

All participants regarded the workshops as a valuable team learning experience. It was felt that the workshops were particularly successful in providing them with a better understanding of other team members' professional roles:

> I now have a better understanding of each others roles, and a better appreciation of the other professionals. (CPN)

The workshops were also considered useful in allowing both CMHTs to share their different professional viewpoints and perspectives:

> The workshops allowed me to hear different professional opinions and to share information with other team members. (occupational therapist)

In addition, participants valued the workshops for providing them with an opportunity to collectively reflect upon their work:

> [The workshops] give you valuable space to reflect on practice. (social worker)

In general, participants appreciated the facilitator's input into the workshops. It was felt that the facilitator ensured the team learning experience was both interesting and enjoyable.

However, there was some feeling that the workshops did not provide enough time for teams to discuss, in sufficient depth, the complex range of issues linked to collaboration. Consequently, it was felt that the sessions tended to be focused more on *'general issues ... rather than particulars'* (psychiatrist). For some, this general focus generated a perception that some of the workshop content overlapped with previous training they had undertaken. Many participants felt the workshops would have been more effective if they had been reduced into a one-day course instead of replacing three of their weekly team meetings.

In addition, there was general concern that so few psychiatrists and psychologists took part in the workshops. For some, this non-attendance undermined the potential value of the workshops as a shared team learning experience. There was also a feeling that the administrative staff should have attended the workshops.

Three-month perspective

The follow-up interviews revealed that participants continued to value the workshops for providing them with a useful team learning experience. After three months, both teams maintained their positive view of the workshops: they were helpful in allowing them to discuss, debate and clarify their collaborative work:

> They [the workshops] provided us with more awareness of the issues linked to working together as an integrated team. (CPN)

Participants also continued to value the workshops in offering them shared reflection time, away from the pressures of their working day:

> The nature of our work makes it is difficult to sit back and reflect, you know what has gone right and wrong and how would you do that differently, the sessions were good in giving us this reflection time. (CPN)

Similarly, participants maintained their positive view of the facilitator's input during the three workshops.

However, the weekly format of the workshops was further questioned. There was a continued agreement that the workshops should have been condensed into a *'focused one day session'* (social worker) instead of replacing three of their regular team meetings.

Although participants valued the workshop information packs, many reported that pressures of work meant that they had little time to read any of the suggested preparatory material contained in their workshop packs. To overcome this problem, it was felt that reading time should be built into the workshops.

Participants in both teams maintained their view that the sessions tended to deal with general issues of collaboration rather than individual team issues. It was felt that more targeted training was needed:

> [The workshops should have been] more relevant to our work, more focused real life problem solving. (social worker)

Participants also continued to feel that the poor attendance of the medical staff needed attention as it would affect their ability to work as an effective CMHT:

> There was a big absence in terms of the doctors, we can't work without them as a team. (social worker)

In addition, participants continued to stress the need to involve both the psychologists and administrative staff in the workshops.

While participants agreed that action planning workshop was a valuable team activity, it was conceded that none of their plans had, so far, been implemented. It was generally felt that heavy workloads were the main cause for their failure to implement the action plans. A few participants suggested that a fourth workshop, offered a few months after the third, could help overcome this problem. In addition, one participant felt that a senior manager should attend the action planning session to ensure they had the necessary support to operationalise their action plans.

Discussion

All participants considered that the workshops have been a valuable team-based learning experience. In general, it was felt that the workshops offered both teams with a useful opportunity to discuss and clarify aspects of their joint team practice. The workshops were also valued in providing both CMHTs with time to reflect upon their interprofessional teamwork. In addition, participants felt all sessions were well facilitated with a range of useful teambuilding activities.

However, it was found that participants' views of the collaboration in their teams did not noticeably alter from pre- to post-workshop. This finding is understandable when one considers that collective team practice is unlikely to change significantly within such a space of time. Nevertheless, it was encouraging to note that the questionnaire data did reveal that participants' understanding of their own role in the team did improve slightly following the workshops.

The poor attendance of medical and psychological staff was problematic. Despite invitations from the both team managers, no psychologists and only two psychiatrists participated. Certainly, the non-attendance of any team member means that training designed for teambuilding is likely to be less effective. It is unclear why these staff failed to attend. Data collected from the two psychiatrists in North Team indicated that both enjoyed the workshops and both actively participated in team discussions. Further work is therefore required to explore how attendance of these staff could be improved in future. In relation to this issue, many participants felt that administrative staff should also attend the workshops. It is unclear why these staff did not attend. Clearly, as members of a CMHT, it would be advantageous for this group of staff to participate.

Despite regarding the action planning exercise in third workshop as an important activity for developing collaboration, the follow-up data revealed that neither team had implemented their plans. Heavy work-loads were cited as the reason for this failure. This is unfortunate. Without ongoing support for this type of activity, it is unlikely to occur within teams working under this type of pressure. This is where management commitment is crucial. Teams need to be given time and space away from their work to achieve any goals relating from an action planning session. This will ensure that their ideas to enhance interprofessional collaboration can be embedded into practice.

Participants voiced a number of concerns about the content and format of the workshops. While most valued the workshops, it was felt that their focus was too broad. This finding is interesting. As noted above, the facilitator negotiated the content of each workshop with both teams before beginning work. It is unclear therefore why participants did not raise their concerns about the content of the workshops when given this opportunity to do so.

In addition, participants found work commitments meant that they had little time to read any of the material on their reading lists before attending the workshops. As indicated, this lack of preparatory reading resulted in superficial discussions in the second workshop. This may have attributed to both the perceived repetition of these workshops with previous training and the feeling that the workshop content was focused on general rather than specific issues of collaboration.

Another concern voiced by participants was linked to the weekly format of the workshops. For many, it was felt that offering the workshops in place of their weekly business meeting meant that they lost important team time. To resolve this issue, it was felt that the three workshops could be condensed into a one-day training session. Given the input of the team managers into the development of these workshops this reaction is surprising as both considered that this format offered the most efficient use of team time. In addition, the issue of 'lost team time' is interesting. Clearly, to reap any benefits from team-based interprofessional education, some commitment of time is necessary. Changing the format of the workshops from two-hour weekly sessions into a one-day course would not alter this issue: the same amount of time is required for both formats.

Collectively, these findings appear to provide some evidence of a possible tension related to this type of team-based learning. Despite valuing their time in the workshops discussing and clarifying issues around collaboration, participants felt inhibited to fully engage with them due to heavy workloads. This tension may have been an important factor in shaping participants' views of the workshops. Indeed, the perceived problems connected to the content and format of the workshops could well be entwined with this tension.

Conclusions

Overall, the workshops were highly valued for providing teams with an opportunity to discuss, clarify and reflect upon issues related to collaboration. The evaluation also revealed a number of areas where the workshops should be developed in future (e.g. ensuring that team action plans are implemented, increasing the attendance of all team members) before they could be offered to other CMHTs.

Importantly, this evaluation revealed that heavy workloads inhibited many participants from fully engaging in this type of work-based learning. This problem appeared to generate a tension within the two teams that undermined their views of the workshops. Educationalists and managers need to be aware of this factor when planning future team-based learning. Further research is also required to explore, in more depth, the effect of this tension on the processes and outcomes of work-based interprofessional education.

Acknowledgements

I would like to thank the members from the two community mental health teams who participated in this work. I would also like to thank Miriam Byfield, Guy Davies, Della Freeth, Sally Glen, Josephine Guerrero, Keith Harris, Joe Herzberg, Tony Leiba, Soo Moore and Gill Williams for their contributions to this project.

This project was jointly funded by grants from the former City and East London Education Confederation and the London Department of Postgraduate Medical and Dental Education.

References

Brown, B, Crawford, P and Darongkamas, J (2000) Blurred Roles and Permeable Boundaries: the Experience of Multidisciplinary Working in Community Mental Health. *Health and Social Care in the Community*, **8**, 425–35.

Brown, S (2000) Outcomes Analysis of a Pain Management for Two Rural Hospitals. *Journal of Nursing Care and Quality*, **14**, 28–34.

Cook, J, Jonikas, J and Razzano, L (1995) A Randomized Evaluation of Consumer vs Non-consumer Training of State Mental Health Service Providers. *Community Mental Health Journal*, **31**, 229–37.

Department of Health (1996) *The Spectrum of Care: Local Services for People with Mental Health Problems*. London: HMSO.

Department of Health (1997) *Developing Partnerships in Mental Health*. London: HMSO.

Department of Health (1998) *Modernising Mental Health Services*. London: HMSO.

Department of Health (2000) *A Health Service of all the Talents: Developing the NHS Workforce*. London: HMSO.

Department of Health and Social Security (1980) *Organisation and Management Problems of Mental Illness Hospitals: Report of a Working Group*. London: HMSO.

Donat, D, Mckeegan, G and Neal, B (1991) Training Inpatient Psychiatric Staff in the use of Behavioural Methods: A Program to Enhance Utilisation. *Psychosocial Rehabilitation Journal*, **15**, 69–74.

Falconer, J, Roth, E, Sutin, J, Strasser, D and Chang, R (1993) The Critical Path Method in Stroke Rehabilitation: Lessons from an Experiment in Cost Containment and Outcome Improvement. *Quarterly Review Bulletin*, **19**, 8–16.

Hammersley, M and Atkinson, P (1995) *Ethnography: Principles in Practice*, (2nd edn). London: Routledge.

Hunter, M and Love, C (1996) Total Quality Management and the Reduction of Inpatient Violence and Costs in a Forensic Psychiatric Hospital. *Psychiatric Services*, **47**, 751–4.

Koppel, I, Barr, H, Reeves, S, Freeth, D and Hammick, M (2001) Establishing a Systematic Approach to Evaluating the Effectiveness of Interprofessional Education. *Issues in Interdisciplinary Care*, **3**, 41–9.

Long, S (1996) Primary Health Care Team Workshop: Team Members' Perspectives. *Journal of Advanced Nursing*, **23**, 935–41.

4

Partnerships in Interprofessional Education and Practice: The Development of a Masters Programme in Interprofessional Practice

Philippa Sully

Introduction

Nationally and internationally, governments and service providers are increasingly recognising the extent and consequences of violence – both intentional and unintentional – domestic violence, rape, torture, suicide, road traffic collisions, transport disasters and violence in institutions and the workplace. Violence causes enormous human cost to individuals, families and society. These issues have raised awareness of the need for interdisciplinary approaches to the care of survivors of violence, as their difficulties can often go unrecognised by health and social care services and employers (Hoff and Adamowski, 1998).

Violence is a manifestation of inequities in power and as such, is a health care as well as a social and political issue. It is a major global health hazard (World Health Organisation, 2002), but relatively little emphasis is put in nursing curricula on caring for survivors (Ross *et al.*, 1998). The reasons for this can only be speculated upon. However, nurses work in an arena where health care practitioners seem reluctant to ask women about their experiences of domestic violence, or to share information with police services involved in the care and safety of survivors (Greenaway *et al.*, 2001).

Because violence pervades all aspects of society, it is not possible to put it and its consequences in terms of care for survivors, in one or two specific domains/disciplines. Recognition of this is crucial when looking at policy and service development, as well as education programmes for the professions involved. Practitioners need to become very skilled at developing relationships with colleagues in other disciplines, in order that they are able to straddle the limits of professional domains, as opposed to staying rigidly within their own disciplines.

However, the paradox is that violence by its very nature violates boundaries. It is therefore important to address this pervasiveness by ensuring in practice, that professional parameters are crossed in an informed and respectful way. This was the case with the development and implementation of this Masters programme.

This chapter examines the development and implementation of an Interprofessional Master of Science programme for practitioners who work with survivors of intentional and unintentional violence. It was developed in an arena of increasing awareness of client need and practitioner vulnerability to violence – both personal in the course of their duties (Little, 1999), but also among the communities they serve. It will address the strategies used to develop, implement and evaluate the nterprofessional MSc: Society, Violence and Practice. It will also explore the partnerships and systems, which evolved and were maintained to support this process.

Background

In October 2000, the European Declaration of Human Rights was enshrined in English Law (*Human Rights Act 1998*). The debate surrounding this and the impact it is having on survivors of violence – as well as those accused of breaking the law – has coincided with the political emphasis and current UK Government policy on promoting partnership in the development and delivery of health and social services in the

United Kingdom both in the voluntary and statutory sectors (*Crime and Disorder Act 1998*, Department of Health, 1999a,b, 2000; MacPherson, 1999; NHS Executive, 1998, 1999, 2000).

As Human Rights cross practice limits and international frontiers, there has been increasing recognition – politically and socially – of the need to work in partnership to co-ordinate the care of survivors across national borders and professional boundaries. These factors have resulted in new developments in the delivery of services to the community and the organisational structures supporting them. A sound example of this is the establishment in the United Kingdom of Multi-Agency Public Protection Panels for the monitoring of sex and violent offenders.

This programme has been developed in the international academic, social and health care arena. The curriculum is based on an outline written by Dr Lee Ann Hoff, a well-recognised specialist in crisis care, and colleagues from the University of Massachusetts, Lowell, USA. Dr Hoff has also worked closely with Prof. Jose Ornelas who has led a similar programme in the Insituto de Psicologia Applicada in Lisbon, Portugal. At the time of writing, programmes are also being developed in Boston and Toronto.

The author is a member of the Department of Applied Psych-social Sciences – all members of which are qualified to higher degree level in disciplines other than nursing and midwifery. This enabled her to gain access to specialists in the field outside as well as within other schools in the University, through the support of her colleagues.

Within this arena, City University in London established this interprofessional programme, which focuses on the delivery of expert practice in caring for survivors of violence of all sorts. Its aim therefore is:

> To develop expert practice in service delivery, research, consultancy and education to survivors of violence and their communities.

The speed in which it was implemented from the first discussions to the first intake of students is a tribute to the commitment of all those involved to services for survivors and thus the development of the programme.

Partnership and authority

Partnership and authority have been integral to the development and successful implementation of this course. Authority is defined by

Obholzer (1994a: 39) as:

> The right to make an ultimate decision, and in an organization it refers to the right to make decisions which are binding on others.

The use of authority within partnerships has ensured that support for the programme's development was available in a number of different professions.

Initially, the author discussed informally the possibility of developing an interprofessional programme with an Inspector in Sector Policing in the Metropolitan Police Service. Sector policing is focused on local communities and the Inspector has sound understanding of the needs of a diverse community.

The Inspector's view was that the course would meet a need in police services for a practise-based programme, which would also have academic standing. However, she recommended that a more senior officer in the Service with more authority than herself, would be the appropriate person with whom to discuss the idea with a view to its relevance and development. The senior officer would be in a position to enable colleagues to contribute to the programme's development by direct involvement or indirectly, by facilitating the development of strategic networks.

In order to submit a formal proposal to their respective senior managers, they wrote a joint report together for them. This collaboration meant that from the start they had to negotiate the use of professional language in order to ensure all parties understood what was proposed and its value.

Consequently the Inspector, her Superintendent, the author's Head of Department and the author, met to discuss the value of the course and how it might be developed. The Superintendent put the author in touch with practitioners and experts in policing, police training, as well as those in other statutory organisations and the voluntary sector. This meant that she was able to work closely with senior staff who had the power to initiate and/or support the development of the programme, line managers who could directly influence practice and practitioners who were interested in caring for survivors of violence and their loved ones.

In accordance with University Ordinances a Course Advisory Board and a Course Management Team were established. Both had representatives from all these service levels. This ensured support in practice for the course development, as well as keeping it grounded in the daily work of practitioners in a variety of disciplines.

The significance of interprofessional collaboration – partnership – became clear when the course content was developed. The timeframe for the submission of the complete MSc programme was short. Feedback and comments were needed quickly, which put pressure on contributors. But it also demonstrated commitment to diverse views by having clear evidence of different perspectives in the course documentation. Partnership was evident in the soliciting and inclusion of comments from contributors in different disciplines.

The process of developing the triggers – as well as all the BSc(Hons) and MSc content – was also interprofessional. The issues raised and dynamics of the discussion in the Course Management Team were very similar to those raised in the classroom, both in enquiry-based and expert-led workshops held by the time of writing.

Strategies and structures

The focus of this programme is the development of practice. The overall strategy used to develop the course was therefore always to keep inter-professional practice in the forefront of every decision. An example of this is the recent decision to make minor amendments to the modules dealing with legal issues and longer term care of survivors (the Legal Response to Intentional and Unintentional Violence and Beyond Crisis), in order to share learning with the MSc on Civil Emergency Management currently being developed by the Department of Adult Nursing in the School.

The Course Advisory Board and the Curriculum Management Team were essential structures underpinning the development of this MSc. Multidisciplinary membership of these committees was established from the outset. This meant that the focus on the broadest aspects of practice was maintained. Disciplines such as the police, the voluntary sector, health care professionals, service providers and educationalists, were represented. Shared responsibility for strategic planning, curriculum development and implementation, was thus ensured. From the beginning it was crucial to avoid meetings being dominated by one professional group.

This was achieved by differentiating between process that promoted the development of team cohesion and anti-task processes such as pairing or fight–flight (Bion, 1961) when chairing meetings and facilitating interdisciplinary workshops. These processes occurred, for example, when discussion was vociferous between two members (pairing) who had shared or had had differing perspectives on an issue that was related to but not part of the task at hand, or when particularly significant cases in individuals' professional practice were explored by the group (fight/ flight). These discussions were often ways in which group members developed their group cohesion through negotiating their roles and deciding their contributions to the task – the process Tuckman (1965) described as 'storming'. These processes mirrored interprofessional practice with survivors and, in the author's experience, were integral to the development of effective working relationships and thus the programme.

The initial stages of programme development were kept low key. This was to ensure the successful implementation of the first two modules with the minimum of disruption to the Departmental and School work-load and that of partners in other disciplines. These modules were offered at BSc(Hons) level and were validated through an existing degree pathway. They were run between July 2000 and March 2001. In effect they turned out to be a successful pilot for the development and imple-mentation of the Masters programme. This strategy ensured that struc-tures, systems, content and its delivery could be examined and developed for the validation of the MSc, which was achieved in March 2001.

Triangular relationships

The establishment of a triangular or three-pronged approach to programme development, ensured a stable base for supporting its devel-opment and implementation. Triangular structures, while ensuring secure bases for systems and developments, can by their very stability, also ensure that once systems are established, they may be very difficult to alter particularly if they become used as an organisational defence (Mattinson, 1980). The possibility of this is kept in mind by the Course Leader when obstructing situations arise that seem impervious to change.

A creative and supportive triangle was that provided by the involve-ment of senior management, line managers and practitioners at the service frontline. Senior managers helped ensure that the authority for supporting and implementing policy changes and decisions was estab-lished. Line managers were able to share the views of their staff as well as influence practice at the 'coalface' while the involvement of practi-tioners ensured the issues in day-to-day practice were not forgotten. This ensured that the course stayed grounded in care of survivors and their communities and in the needs of staff to provide the services. This structure ensured that the strategic and practical approaches needed to implement the programme were addressed.

As the course has evolved it has become clear that the University forms an integral part of a number of triangles. Some examples are:

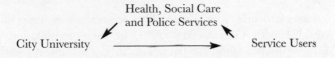

The charity Refuge provides classroom space for the course and their staff have been actively involved formally and informally in its development, City University provides the academic services and validation of the programme while the students are the raison d'etre of the course, as they will take new learning into practice.

Health, Social Care
and Police Services

City University   ——————→   Service Users

Here the academic institution provides teaching, research backup and validation to student experiences in their work in the statutory and voluntary sectors, who in turn work with service users in the community.

Interprofessional practice MSc: society, violence and practice

Koppel *et al.* (2001) in their review of research into interprofessional education, suggest that this is best done on continuing professional development programmes. They also suggest that it is more successful in achieving the expected outcomes if the programme is of a longer rather than shorter duration. This MSc programme is for experienced practitioners and therefore constitutes continuing professional development, which can be completed within two to five years.

Although modules may be taken as stand alone courses, it is recommended that students pursue the entire programme for it to have the maximum benefit to their professional development and care delivery.

Student selection

As the degree programme is about practice and its development, students are required to have at least 2 years' post-qualifying experience in working with survivors. A first degree is not required, but successful applicants must demonstrate:

the relevance of the degree to their own practice development
the ability to study at master's level.

All shortlisted applicants are interviewed. This is a departure from established School policy for Masters programmes and initially caused some problems with admissions systems. One of the main reasons for deciding to interview prospective students was that some course content was of necessity likely to be distressing and where possible it was important to discuss face-to-face the likely effects this might have.

Course structure

The course structure is modular. This framework is supported by the World Health Organisation (2002) in their consultation paper for Masters programme in the field. Two modules are run together so students spend approximately one day a fortnight in class.

The programme consists of a total of eight modules, one of which is compulsory and another optional. They can be taken as stand-alone courses or as part of an MSc in Interprofessional Practice in the School's Continuing Professional Development Programme. The compulsory module for all these programmes is 'Partnership in Practice'. In autumn 2001 it was run alongside the module 'Emergency and Crisis Responses to Victims of Violence'.

Modules

Partnership in practice (compulsory module)

This module gives practitioners the opportunity to study together in a flexible but structured way, enabling them to share learning. It mirrors the innovative and creative ways of working for partners in practice, as outlined in: *A Health Service of all the Talents* (Department of Health, 2000).

The aims of this module are:

To evaluate interagency policies and strategies for the promotion of interprofessional practice.
To examine critically intergroup interests and their effect on interprofessional practice at all levels.

To reflect upon the impact of interprofessional working in the students' own areas with a view to advancing practice.

To examine critically the influence of ethics, human rights legislation and research on partnership in practice. (City University, 2001)

Content delivery is through a mixture of interprofessional seminars and experiential learning. The focus is the relationships and communication in the group and in the individual processes inherent in experiential workshops, how they are explained by theory and research and their relevance in practice. These explorations provide opportunities to explore and practice further the skills necessary for effective interprofessional working. The Reflective Practice sessions at the end of each study day, provide students with time to explore communication within and across disciplines, using incidents from their own practice.

Its focus is the dynamics of conscious and unconscious processes in working across professional boundaries. Content delivery is largely experiential with workshops addressing communication, teamwork, group process as well as the task focus and evidence base for effective interprofessional practice. Reflection on and the development of practice is integral to this module as indeed it is for this entire MSc programme.

Emergency and crisis responses to victims of violence

Prevention, Public Education and Community Organisation
Historical, Social and Cultural Perspectives on Violence and Abuse
The Legal Response to Intentional and Unintentional Violence
Beyond Crisis: Psychosocial Services for Survivors of Violence
Elective Placement (Optional – students can replace this with a module
   from other MSc's)
Research Methods
Research Thesis

Study Hours per Module:

12 Taught Hours
20 Reflective Practice Hours
68 Self-directed hours
Total Credits: 120 at Masters level (QAA standards) (under review)

Ultimately the hope is that the module: The Legal Response to Intentional and Unintentional Violence will be delivered on the internet.

Staff in an Australian University, which is closely affiliated to the local Police Academy, are keen to be involved in the web-based development of this module. This would enable students in different parts of the world to study and work together in a flexible manner despite differences in time culture and geography. As violence is an issue affecting the quality of life of people around the world, it is argued that an interactive web-based module would go some way to bridge barriers of understanding, language, culture and law in order to deliver effective services to survivors.

Content delivery

As the programme is grounded in practice, its delivery focuses on the development of skills in working across disciplines as well as the development of the evidence-base for practice. Too often services to survivors fail because communication across disciplines and services has been inadequate. For this reason Enquiry-based Learning (EBL) and other interactive ways of learning were chosen for the delivery of much of the content. These methods also promote choice, autonomy in learning and reflection – skills which are integral to sound interprofessional practice.

Rigidly prescribing content, limits choice and can be disempowering, as well as stifling of creativity in application to the issues at hand. This stultifying experience can be readily seen in survivors of violence who can be disabled from taking initiative or control (Mullender, 1996). The course developers obviously wanted to avoid this consequence of violence being mirrored in classroom processes.

Students are experienced practitioners from a variety of disciplines. They therefore bring diverse skills and understanding to the course content. The richness of classroom experience is in the different perspectives they bring to the same content. They are encouraged to learn together in a structured but flexible manner, working across disciplines as a group or partnership. An interprofessional approach is also described as being essential to the success of EBL (Long *et al.*, 1999). The use of case scenarios, issues or 'triggers' allows for a framework of enquiry in which participants can work collaboratively and share their different expertise on the issues raised.

In the modules using EBL, interprofessional workshops were arranged. These were led by two or more experts in their fields of working with survivors such as accident and emergency staff, police officers, clinical psychologists and researchers and chaired by the author, usually with the assistance of a colleague. These provided an immediate example of collaboration despite differing priorities and perspectives.

Assessment

Each module has a summative assessment. In order to keep to the focus of practice development, all assessments are grounded in practice. Students may negotiate their assignments with the teaching staff responsible.

As this programme deals with painful and anxiety-provoking issues, the emotions they might elicit can become manifest in abusive group processes (Halton, 1994). Lecturers can be perceived unconsciously as holding the power to the students' success. Care is therefore taken that assessment is not used as a way of abusing power, for example, by refusing to renegotiate assignments with students.

Systems, containment and reflection

Support

Reflection on practice is an integral part of the course and its delivery. Boud *et al.* (1985) describe a model of reflection, which underpins the approach used by the co-facilitators of the course. Students have an hour of group supervision on each study day for each module. This is to allow them the opportunity to reflect on and develop their practice. They are required to keep reflective journals, which provide the foundation for this work.

Sound facilitation by two lecturers is used to ensure psychological safety. This is crucial if abusive group processes – the dark side of the human psyche (Guerrero and Anderson, 1998) are to be kept to the minimum in the learning process. The importance of providing clear boundaries such as working to the negotiated group contract, keeping to time limits and using the same classroom space is integral to this. Psychological safety is also an essential feature of working with survivors and therefore needs to be experienced in the classroom, as clearly established parameters for practice are crucial in ensuring survivors receive sensitive and appropriate care.

The education institution needs also to be able to contain the anxieties raised by delivering a course of this type (Obholzer, 1994b). There is also the risk of abusive systems being established within the organisation delivering the education or care services (Moylan, 1994).

Therefore it is possible that lecturers might experience what many survivors and practitioners in the field of violence experience – that is, the parallel process of being the abused by the system in which they work (Hawkins and Shohet, 1989; Proctor, 1994). Therefore all the module leaders are required to attend their own group supervision with a qualified psychotherapist. This strategy was established in order to ensure safe practice in the classroom as well as in the field.

Challenges in the system

What is significant about the programme's development and implementation is that the parallel processes so evident in the practice of the human services (Obholzer and Roberts, 1994), are also evident here. Challenges were not always readily foreseeable, or indeed, when they were envisaged the difficulties were not necessarily prevented.

The Continuing Professional Development framework was undergoing change at the time the MSc was being implemented. Support systems were not able to adapt to the changing nature of the requirements of this interprofessional programme. This change in working practices coincided with the School of Nursing and Midwifery having to deal with inquiries from disciplines as diverse as policing and voluntary work. This meant that despite agreements, new or changed documentation this was not always achieved in time, or used. That shortlisted applicants were interviewed, caused difficulties because this was not necessarily the process for established Masters programmes. Problems were exacerbated because authority for supporting change was invested in different departments.

Sensitivity to people's working practices needed to be balanced with the determination to establish and run the programme. Careful negotiation was necessary at times to ensure the introduction of new approaches in order to support this programme.

Containment and clarification

Throughout the development and delivery of the course, the major challenges have been the clarification of language and maintaining boundaries.

The manner in which language is used differently by different disciplines has been evident throughout this project. Clarification of terminology has been essential to avoid misunderstandings. The use of metaphor is an example of this – other disciplines might not understand what a police officer means by a 'toolkit'.

At times, ensuring that boundaries were kept during meetings, in class and in supervision was demanding. Observing time limits, keeping task-focused and working to agreed agendas rather than be sidelined by discussing other issues, have required skilful facilitation. This has been necessary to ensure less confident members have been encouraged to offer their opinions, sensitive topics are addressed and processes in supervision have not been avoided.

The importance of addressing process and keeping to the task has become manifest in these workshops. Roberts (1994) identifies how Bion's ideas of basic assumptions in group process can deflect practitioners from the task of addressing painful issues and thus not keep to the task of providing services to those in need. By establishing a constant and secure relationship (Bowlby, 1988, chap. 8) with the students through the allocation of personal tutors and co-facilitation throughout the course, lecturers are able to acknowledge and address with students difficult processes, which are the inevitable consequence of dealing with these painful and destructive aspects of human experience (see Stevenson, 1994).

Programme evaluation

In line with suggestions offered by Koppel *et al.* (2001), in order to form a base line for the impact of this programme on student learning and practice the programme is being evaluated concurrent with its delivery. The Research Fellow in the Department has carried out before and after discussions with students on the BSc(Hons) modules, and has held follow-up interviews with some of them. Using semi-structured focus groups and reflective writing he is also evaluating the MSc programme.

Student feedback has been largely positive with students having indicated how their awareness and practice have changed and developed. They are describing:

increasing ability to apply theory to practice;
enhanced awareness of the evidence base for their interprofessional practice with survivors of violence;
increased knowledge and skill about working with survivors of violence.

Conclusion

This MSc preceded the World Health Organisation's report on the need for an interprofessional course on global injury prevention (WHO, 2002). The report emphasises the need for flexible interprofessional learning, which is fundamental to the City University programme.

That this course led the way in this field and was developed in such a short time, is a tribute to the dedication of all those involved. They have been willing to face some difficult processes in their commitment to improving the service to survivors of violence, through the establishment of this innovative programme.

The interprofessional focus with the aim of developing practice in its broadest sense, has according to students' reports to date, been successful. It has been an honour to work with such courageous people.

References

Boud, D, Keogh, R, and Walker, D (1985) *Turning Reflection into Learning*. London: Kogan Page.

Bion, W R (1961) *Experiences with Groups: and other papers*. London: Tavistock.

Bowlby, J (1988) *A Secure Base*, chap. 8. London: Tavistock/Routledge.

City University (2001) *Partnership in Practice. Curriculum Documents*. London: City University.

Department of Health (1999a) *Making a Difference*. London: Department of Health.

DOH (1999b) *Modernising Health and Social Services National Priorities Guidance 2000/01–2002/03*. London: Department of Health.

DOH (2000) *A Health Service of all the Talents: Developing the NHS Workforce*. London: Department of Health.

Greenaway, K, Sully, P, and Reeves (2001) The Suppression of Murder. *Police Review,12 October*, **109**(5643), 26–8.

Guerrero, L K and Anderson, P A (1998) The Dark Side of Jealousy and Envy: Desire, Delusion, Desperation, and Destructive Communication, chap. 2 in Spitzberg, B H and Cupach, W R (eds) *The Dark Side of Close Relationships*. New Jersey: LEA Publishers.

Halton (1994) Some Unconscious Aspects of Organizational Life: Contributions from Psychoanalysis, chap. 1 in Obholzer, A and Roberts, V Z (eds) *The Unconscious at Work. Individual and Organizational Stress in the Human Services*. London: Routledge.

Hawkins, P and Shohet, R (1989) *Supervision in the Helping Professions*. Milton Keynes: Oxford University Press.

Home Office (1998) *The Crime and Disorder Act 1998*. London: Home Office.

Home Office (1998) *The Human Rights Act 1998*. London: Home Office.

Hoff, L A and Adamowski, K (1998) *Creating Excellence in Crisis Care*. San Francisco: Jossey-Bass.

Koppel, I, Barr, H, Reeves, S, Freeth, D, and Hammick, M (2001) Establishing a Systematic Approach to Evaluating the Effectiveness of Interprofessional Education. *Issues in Interdisciplinary Care*, **3**(1) January 2001, 41–9.

Little, L (1999) Risk factors for Assaults on Nursing Staff: Childhood Abuse and Educational Level. *Journal of Nursing Administration, December*, **29**(12), 22–9.

Long, G, Grandis, S, Glasper, E A (1999) Investing in Practice: Enquiry- and Problem-based Learning. *British Journal of Nursing, 1999*, **8**(17), 1171–74.

Macpherson, W (1999) *The Stephen Lawrence Inquiry*, Vol. 1 & 2. London: The Home Office.

Mattinson, J (1981) *The Deadly Equal Triangle* in Change and Renewal in Psychodynamic Social Work: British and American Developments Practice and Education for Services to Families and Children. Massachusetts/London: Smiths College School of Social Work/Group for the Advancement of Psychotherapy in Social Work.

Moylan, D (1994) The Dangers of Contagion Projective Identification Processes in Institutions, chap. 5 in Obholzer, A and Roberts, V Z (eds) *The Unconscious at Work. Individual and Organizational Stress in the Human Services*. London: Routledge.

Mullender, A (1996) *Rethinking Domestic Violence*. London: Routledge.

National Health Service Executive (1996) *Education and Training Planning Guidance*. London: HMSO.

NHS Executive (1998) *The New NHS, Modern and Dependable: a National Framework for Assessing Performance*, Consultation Document. London: NHS Executive.

NHS Executive (1999) *Working Together. Securing a Quality Workforce for the NHS*. London: Department of Health.

NHS Executive (2000) *The NHS Plan*. London: Department of Health.

Obholzer, A (1994a) Authority, Power and Leadership. Contributions from Group Relations Training, chap. 4 in Obholzer, A and Roberts, V Z (eds) *The Unconscious at Work. Individual and Organizational Stress in the Human Services*. London: Routledge.

Obholzer, A (1994b) Managing Social Anxieties in Public Sector Organizations, chap. 18 in Obholzer, A and Roberts, V Z (eds) *The Unconscious at Work. Individual and Organizational Stress in the Human Services*. London: Routledge.

Obholzer, A and Roberts, V Z (1994) *he Troublesome Individual and the Troubled Institution*, chap. 14 in Obholzer, A and Roberts, V Z (eds) The *Unconscious at Work. Individual and Organizational Stress in the Human Services*. London: Routledge.

Øvretveit, J (1993) *Co-ordinating Community Care: Multidisciplinary Teams and Care Management*. Buckingham: Oxford University Press.

Proctor, B (1994) Supervision – Competence, Confidence, Accountability. *British Journal of Guidance and Counselling*, **22**(3), 309–18.

Reeves, S (2000) Community-based Interprofessional Education for Medical, Nursing and Dental Students. *Health and Social Care in the Community*, **8**, 269–76.

Reeves, S (2001) A Systematic Review of the Effects of Interprofessional Education on Staff Involved in the Care of Adults with Mental Health Problems. *Journal of Psychiatric Mental Health Nursing*, **8**, 533–42.

Reeves, S and Freeth, D (2002) The London Training Ward: an Innovative Interprofessional Learning Initiative. *Journal of Interprofessional Care*, **16**, 41–52.

Roberts, V Z (1994) Conflict and Collaboration Managing Intergroup Relations, chap. 20 in Obholzer, A and Roberts, V Z (eds) *The Unconscious at Work. Individual and Organizational Stress in the Human Services.* London: Routledge.

Ross, M M, Hoff, L A, and Coutu-Wakulczyk, G (1998) Nursing Curricula and Violence Issues. *Journal of Nursing Education*, **37**(2), 53–60.

Rutter, D and Hagart, J (1990) Alcohol Training in South-East England: A Survey and Evaluation. *Alcohol & Alcoholism*, **25**(6), 699–709.

Sainsbury Centre for Mental Health (1997) Pulling *Together: the Future Roles and Training of Mental Health Staff.* London: Sainsbury Centre for Mental Health.

Stein, J and Brown, S (1995) 'All in this Together': an Evaluation of Joint Training on the Abuse of Adults with Learning Disabilities. *Health and Social Care in the Community*, **3**, 205–14.

Stevens, L, Kinmouth, A, Peveler, R and Thompson, C (1997) The Hampshire Depression Project: Development and Piloting of Clinical Practice Guidelines and Education About Depression in Primary Health Care. *Medical Education*, **31**, 375–9.

Stevenson, O (1994) Child Protection: Where now for Interprofessional Work? chap. 7 in Leathard, A (ed.) *Going Interprofessional. Working Together for Health and Welfare.* London: Routledge.

Tuckman, B W (1965) Developmental Sequence in Small Groups. *Psychological Bulletin*, **63**, 384–99.

World Health Organisation (2002) *Report on the Consultation for the Development of a Global Injury Prevention Curriculum and Training Course.* Geneva: World Health Organisation.

5

Interprofessional Practice Teacher Education

Dave Sims and Kate Leonard

Introduction

This chapter will describe and evaluate a model of interprofessional post-qualifying education developed to meet the learning needs of practice teachers who support students on social work and community nursing qualifying programmes. The Interprofessional Practice Teacher Course, which has been delivered at South Bank University since 1997, developed as a result of a national initiative to promote interprofessional training for practice teachers. The course built upon many years experience of providing a uni-professional training programme for social workers.

The chapter will explore the rationale for changing to an interprofessional approach, describe and reflect upon the programme and its development and evaluate the outcomes with reference to an evaluation carried out with former students, their managers and training officers. Key issues which have arisen during the development and implementation of the course will be highlighted, in order to identify lessons learned which could be helpful to those developing future programmes of interprofessional education.

The context of practice teacher education

Practice teachers and clinical supervisors play a key role in the training and socialising of the next generation of health and welfare professionals within the work context. (Bartholemew et al., 1996)

This quotation opens the report of the Joint Practice Teaching Initiative (JPTI), which was an important national development project led jointly by CCETSW, the English National Board for Nursing Midwifery and Health Visiting (ENB), and the College of Occupational Therapy. The project carried out its work between 1990 and 1995, with the aim of promoting and developing joint teaching programmes for practice teachers/clinical supervisors in nursing, social work and occupational therapy. Twelve projects were initiated and funded across the United Kingdom and six jointly validated programmes were run and evaluated in England.

The context of the JPTI was the growing realisation during the 1980s that shared learning and joint training could contribute in some way to improving collaboration and communication between health and social care professionals. A number of child abuse tragedies had focused attention on the need to improve interprofessional collaboration. Additionally, CCETSW and the ENB were already engaged in important work in developing pre-qualifying programmes in learning disability nursing and social work, which were beginning to break the mould of professional training. One such programme was subsequently developed at South Bank University and directly led to the development of the interprofessional practice teaching course which is the subject of this chapter.

The JPTI report in 1995 noted some of the achievements of the project. Two key outcomes were:

- The breaking down of professional barriers. Learning together had meant that participants in joint initiatives had critically examined occupational cultures, values and working practices and come to a better understanding of and greater respect for each other's roles and responsibilities.
- The design and implementation of a Core Curriculum module based on the common ground from the training programmes of the three different professions involved in the project.

The latter outcome clearly demonstrated that some aspects of practice teacher education were generic to different professions, and this provided an important building block for shared learning. This was to be a key principle that would underpin the development of the interprofessional practice teaching course which is the focus of this chapter.

Background and development of the course

Development work began on the Interprofessional Practice Teaching Course in 1997 following a need by the University to change its approach to practice teacher education for social work. This change was necessary for two reasons.

First, the South Bank Practice Teaching Programme run jointly with the Blackfriars Centre had to be reviewed due to a reorganisation of practice learning funding announced by CCETSW. The implication of the change in funding arrangements meant that the Centre's funding would be reduced and that the university would need to take over the resourcing of the then existing practice teacher programme if this were to continue. Although management of the programme had been a collaborative venture it had always been delivered at the Centre, not at the University. In addition, the programme had been designed and delivered exclusively for practice teachers of students on the university postgraduate Diploma in Social Work (DipSW) programme. This had meant that opportunities for shared learning had not been integral to the programme. However, if the programme were to be part of the university provision formally and based in the Faculty of Health, then there would be much greater possibility of shared learning with other professionals in training, especially community nurses and occupational therapists.

The second reason for change was derived from the fact that the practice teaching programme was only designed for social work practice teachers and could therefore not be accessed by nurses who were practice teachers on another social work programme at the University, the joint training programme in learning disability nursing and social work referred to earlier. On this programme it was common and accepted practice that nurses would act as practice teachers to social work students, in line with CCETSW's acceptance that suitably qualified practice teachers from other professional groups could supervise social work students on placement. Ironically though, although recognised as practice teachers for social work students, nurses could not undertake practice teacher training within the university (there was no community nurse practice teacher training offered by the university at this time). Staff running the joint programme were therefore enthusiastic about developing a new programme for practice teachers which would be interprofessional in focus and would enable them to experience some of the same challenges and learning experienced by their students.

Following very positive feedback and evaluation of the joint training programme in learning disability nursing and social work, the University had approached CCETSW to request development funding for an interprofessional practice teaching programme. CCETSW responded positively and the university matched the funding allocated such that sufficient money was available to appoint a development worker.

Learning to support learning

The Interprofessional Practice Teaching Course offers practice teachers from health and social care an opportunity to learn to be practice teachers. This is the core task of the course. The role of the practice teacher is a role with commonalities across professions and so the course offers an opportunity to train teachers, supervisors and mentors of the future in the principles, costs and benefits of interprofessional working. The knowledge base of adult learning, anti-discriminatory practice and interprofessional working and learning together underpin the course. Participants (a term we will use to refer to either community nurse or social work practice teachers on the course) learn about each other's roles and responsibilities as part of the learning environment.

The course is primarily for practice teachers taking students on placement from three programmes at the university, these being a PGDip/BSc Community Nursing Programme, an MA in Social Work and a BSc in Nursing and Social Work studies (Learning Difficulties). Participants are occasionally supervisors of students on other university social work and community nursing courses in London. The course is also recognised by the Occupational Therapy team at the University as meeting the College of Occupational Therapy requirements for practice teachers.

Participants study two units at level three or Masters level on a part-time basis over one academic year. A further additional unit for community nurses was validated and approved by the ENB in 1999. The course was re-approved to meet the new ENB mentor requirements in July 2001 and as a result reduced again to the two core units for all participants. The course was then revalidated in May 2002 to meet the new Nursing and Midwifery Council (NMC) Mentor requirements and to provide a pathway at Masters level to the NMC Practice Educator and Nurse Tutor awards. This followed new guidance issued by the ENB in 2001 (ENB, 2001).

Initially, the course was a stand-alone qualification, but following the changes mentioned above, it was decided to develop a framework within which participants could progress further. Consequently, those practice teachers who study a further two units at Masters level can now gain a Post Graduate Certificate in Interprofessional Practice Education. Pathways have also been created to follow at level three to gain a degree or to study further for a Masters degree in Practice or Teaching and Learning. A key imperative throughout the introduction of these changes has been to preserve the interprofessional core at the heart of these new opportunities for development.

A Programme Management Committee (PMC) oversees the course, which continues to meet the CCETSW (now the General Social Care Council – GSCC) requirements for the Social Work Practice Teacher Award and through one intake per year. The PMC meets three times a year and is made up of representatives from the University, NHS Trusts and Local Authority Social Services Departments. Partner representatives also attend course boards twice a year to review the course progress with representatives of the practice teachers attending the course. The multi-professional composition of the PMC reflects the interprofessional nature of the course.

What is a truly interprofessional course?

This question frequently arises when delivering shared learning. There are many reasons for providing interprofessional education. More recently the political drive for professionals within the health service and workers from the local authority, voluntary and private sector to train and work together has accelerated developments. While certain services such as learning disability and mental health services have been working towards or within 'integrated teams', there is now a more focused approach to piloting pre- and post-qualifying training.

Definitions by the Centre for the Advancement of Interprofessional Education (CAIPE) refer to Interprofessional education as

'Occasions when two or more professions learn from and about each other to improve collaboration and the quality of care'.

Multi-professional education is described as 'Occasions when two or more professions learn side by side for what ever reason'. (cited in Barr, 2002, p. 6)

Qualifying courses at the university offer the experience of interprofessional 'meeting points' in a variety of ways. These include: providing a specific module on interprofessional working; learning together about a particular service user group; studying core disciplines of health and social care such as social policy, professional values, sociology, biology; studying a research methods module; and finally, specific to this chapter, learning about a role common to each profession that is, practice learning and teaching.

Uni-professional, multi-professional, interprofessional?

The course offers aspects of multi- and interprofessional education. But what combinations count when considering the mix of professions involved? If the student group is largely uni-professional (as it was in the first cohort of the course – see Table 5.1) but the lecturing staff are from another profession, does this count? In the first year the practice teachers consisted of many social workers and only two nurses. The community nurse and social work lecturers co-worked together in order to counter balance the emphasis on social work. The lecturers were new to inter-professional working and although we aimed to model interprofessional working we also took strength in meeting the group's needs by offering our different professional perspectives on placement issues for each profession. By doing this we learnt about each others' professional backgrounds and issues for practice teachers.

This opportunity to learn from each other helped us to broaden the range of reading in relation to practice teaching across health, social care and education. There was a need to use a range of interprofessional writing and literature from all professions in order to maintain and model a balance and to demonstrate that the lecturers value each of the professions. We have found that different professions bring different strengths to an interprofessional course. For example, there is more written on reflective practice in the nursing literature than in social work

Table 5.1 Getting the balance right – changes in the student profile

Year intake	Number of participants	Number of social workers	Number of community nurses
1997/98	23	21	2
1998/99	21	15	6
1999/2000	37	19	18
2000/01	32	15	17
2001/02	46	20	26

texts and more written on anti-oppressive practice in social work literature than in nursing texts (although it is important to note that health inequalities are well documented in the nursing literature).

In the delivery of the course the knowledge base of each profession has been explored and debated as part of the transferable learning opportunities available. This has included an exploration of the new NMC (2002) Code of Conduct for nurses and the previous UKCC (1992) Code of Conduct, and the Code of Conduct for social care workers and social care employers just introduced for the first time by the GSCC (2002). Wilmott (1995) has compared the previous code of conduct of the UKCC (1992) and the British Association of Social Workers Code of Ethics for social workers and identifies key areas for discussion relating to the different professions and their rules in respect of society, risk and equalities issues. Discussion of such ideas has provided a basis for lecturers from one profession becoming competent and confident in delivering teaching on particular aspects of the practice learning experience that arc common and comparative to all in health and social care.

Returning to the question posed earlier, how many of each different professional group do you need on a course to call it truly interprofessional? This is very difficult to answer. In terms of this course, there has been an expectation from the qualifying courses for which we were training practice teachers that an even balance of the range of professionals makes a better interprofessional experience. Certainly where there is an expectation of self-directed learning, presentations and sharing in small groups this allows for there to be a balance of opinion, dialogue and debate across and within professional groups. It also avoids a particular profession becoming stereotyped with one or two people representing all social workers or all nurses. However, the answer to the question may be more about attitude and motivation than numbers. Practice teachers who begin the course come with a variety of expectations and a continuum of motivation to learn interprofessionally. The process of attending the course can increase motivation and learning. On the other hand, some practice teachers see the interprofessional context as a side issue that is distracting and as interrupting the core task of learning how to be a practice teacher for a particular profession.

The learning on the course ranges from working together through to how practice teachers can provide practical experiences of interprofessional working to their students in the placement. In order to develop the commitment of practice teachers the expectation now is that applicants for the course sign up to the interprofessional context of the course. This is now explicitly addressed through the application form, where applicants are expected to consider what they wish to gain from such a course. The ground rules agreed at the beginning of the course include a commitment to learning in an interprofessional context. In the teaching sessions we ask practice teachers to take a risk and mingle rather than taking the safe approach of working with others from the same professional background. This mingling is expected *within* the professions as well as *between* professions, for example, children and families social workers could work together but exclude adult social workers, or district nurses might work together but exclude health visitors or social workers.

It is often the case that professionals find they have more in common if they identify the service user group that they work with, for example, district nurses and social workers working with older people. The course encourages the development of understandings based on this principle. It is also expected that interprofessional issues are discussed in the assessed pieces of work. The course therefore encourages participants to look critically at their role and at interprofessional working.

Key challenges as the course has developed

Assessment

The design of learning outcomes and the framework for assessment on an interprofessional course needs to meet the professional requirements of each professional body and meet the university requirements for the academic level being studied. This can be a substantial challenge if not a deterrent to establishing interprofessional developments. What of course, is most helpful, is where the professional bodies are already agreed about the value of shared learning and willing to facilitate the process. This was the case when the course being described here was being proposed.

To devise an appropriate framework for assessment there needs to be a core process of mapping professional outcomes across professional groups and of assimilating University requirements for unit and course outcomes. The skill lies in adapting language so that it is user friendly and transparent in its meaning across professional and academic boundaries. The 'Plain English' principle is a useful one to inform this process. The General Social Care Council now expects documentation to use plain English and avoid jargon. It has been much reported that jargon can be used by professional groups to enhance status, exert power and control towards service users and other professionals and to provide protective barriers to understanding a particular profession. Words such as 'clinical', 'mentorship' and 'supervision' may have different meanings for different professionals, for example. Other words are used by particular professions but not by all, for example, 'audit', 'preceptorship' and 'anti-oppressive practice'. In so far as interprofessional education represents the meeting of different professional cultures, it is important that communication is enhanced between professionals by ensuring terms are clarified and differences understood.

The course validation document and subsequent documentation provided to practice teachers therefore includes a glossary of agreed words with definitions and is written in a generic language. This has made the course and unit outcomes easily transferable for uni- and interprofessional groups across the university so avoiding replication and the need for several different short teaching courses to be validated because the language used in describing them masked their similarities.

How are practice teachers assessed?

A key method of assessment is through the role of the *Practice Assessor*. The course uses direct observation of three practice teaching sessions by an experienced practice assessor of the practice teacher in training. The Practice Assessor will normally be a qualified professional from the same or allied professional group as the practice teacher. It is desirable they hold a teaching award. They will have at least two years' experience of one of the following: practice teaching with at least two students; staff supervision; post-qualifying mentoring; teaching and assessing workers or students. They will also have proven experience of implementing anti-oppressive practice,have an understanding of the characteristics of adult learning and of how adults learn and be familiar with the requirements for professional qualification of the student the practice teacher will be teaching and assessing.

The practice assessor role encompasses a facilitative, teaching role as well as assessor role as there is a need for the assessor to provide specific and ongoing feedback to enable the practice teacher to progress their teaching practice to a competent level by the end of the three observations.

The method of direct observation is used alongside two written academic assignments and a portfolio that includes evidence of assessment reports written by the practice assessor in respect of the practice teacher. The course prioritises regular meetings between the practice teacher and their student as a mechanism for ongoing assessment and support.

These are referred to as 'practice tutorials', as defined by Shardlow and Doel (1996). This recognises the need to ensure a regular formal meeting but does not confuse this with other notions of supervision that mean very different things to each profession. Observation of the practice tutorial by the practice assessor is essential as it offers the only *direct* evidence of the competence of the practice teacher. The other forms of assessment provide indirect evidence and elicit academic ability and the knowledge base that informs the design of learning and teaching opportunities. The practice tutorial signifies the importance of the educational experience and treats this as the prime focus with all the aspects of teaching learning and assessment addressed within this framework. This is a requirement of the GSCC for the assessment of social work practice teachers.

The role of the practice assessor is further explored by Leonard (1998). This role has been developed and applied interprofessionally on this course. Practice teaching competence is assessed under five key headings defined by CCETSW (1996), these being values, management of the placement, teaching, assessment and reflective practice. Because they are recognised as comprehensive, these competencies are used as the requirements for practice teaching for *all* practice teachers on the course, whether nurse or social worker. Each requirement has a number of elements for which sufficient evidence to pass must be provided by the assessor in the form of written reports. The language used is generic and relates to the teaching and assessing role rather than the specific profession. The assessment provided by the assessor is included in the portfolio and their recommendation of a pass/fail mark is considered by the overall marker in the light of all the evidence of competency within the portfolio.

Values in interprofessional practice

Another important aspect in relation to assessment is the development of service user involvement in the training of practice teachers. The involvement of service users in professional education and the assessment of students is now expected by the GSCC for its new Social Work Degree, and service users are becoming more central to the planning and service delivery of the National Health Service (NHS), Local Authority and voluntary sector services in health and social care. Service users have already played an important part in professional training programmes (Davis *et al.*, 1999). Cuming and Wilkins (2000) explore the practicalities of involving service users in assessing social work students and provide helpful guidelines as an appendix. On the course we encourage practice teachers to consider many different methods of assessment in order to provide more holistic and fair evidence of competence. Service user feedback is encouraged in relation to observed, assessed visits by the practice teacher and in reviewing the overall service offered by the student. Practice Teachers of the future should be considering service users' views as formally recognised evidence about their student's performance, alongside other evidence.

Feedback from course participants and other stakeholders

In 2001 an evaluation was carried out by the course team to gain feedback from former practice teachers , their managers and from social work training officers and professional development nurses who had been involved with the course. A survey questionnaire was sent to all previous practice teachers and stakeholders asking for comment on a range of aspects relating to the course and its outcomes. Key questions to practice teachers included; their initial expectations of the course; its impact on their competence as practice teachers and on job prospects, job satisfaction and enhancement; ways in which the course was either helpful or did not take account of their individual needs and circumstances; and whether the interprofessional nature of the course brought with it benefits and if so, what these were. A mixture of open and closed questions were used so that respondents could provide explanations of their individual responses. A total of 27 practice teachers completed a questionnaire, comprising 15 social workers and 12 community nurses. Seven managers and nine training officers also responded.

Practice teachers' expectations of the course

There was striking similarity between the responses of both professional groups about their reasons for undertaking the course. The three most common reasons related to an increase in job prospects, an enhancement of job satisfaction and the opportunity to teach qualifying students. A slightly higher proportion of nurses than social workers also appeared motivated by gaining post-qualifying credits. This may reflect the fact that the post-qualifying framework in the NHS is arguably more strongly established (and certainly better funded) than the social work one, which is about to be reviewed by the GSCC.

Developing competence as a practice teacher – benefits of the course

Practice teachers were asked about the benefits of the course and whether it had increased their competence as either a practice teacher or as a practitioner. Both nurses and social workers cited the value of exploring theoretical perspectives and the value of reflecting on their practice – this was particularly prominent amongst the social workers, two of whom specifically valued the opportunity to question and analyse their practice. 'Reflection' was also cited in other responses by social workers. One Practice Teacher referred to becoming more of a reflective practitioner and another found reflecting on their own practice particularly beneficial. Another said the main benefit from the course was understanding about adult learning and looking again at what they themselves did in their work and what it meant. Coverage of theories of learning and reflection were positively reported.

In these sections of the questionnaire, it was the nurses who more commonly cited the interprofessional benefits, even though the survey contained a later section specifically related to this. Nurses valued the shared training with social workers and found the interprofessional aspect and working with students from other disciplines helpful. Responses common to both the nurses and social workers also included the usefulness of the course in terms of planning a curriculum and training sessions for their own students in practice. Two nurses alluded to an increase in confidence as a result of the course.

Overall, what these responses suggest is that there was a general professional development aspect to the course, which had a similar impact on the two professional groups. Not surprisingly there were a range of individualised responses, but overall an increase in skills appeared to be common across the two groups.

Benefits of the course being run interprofessionally

Again here, practice teachers' responses fell into some areas of consensus. Learning about other professions they networked with and understanding the difficulties of other agencies were benefits cited by nurses. One social worker described a benefit as being the ability to discuss openly and honestly different views and values regarding professions, which helped to break down barriers and give an increased awareness of nursing competencies. Practice teachers from both professions said that learning about the roles and tasks of the other profession had been beneficial. A social worker commented that there were benefits in learning the views of others and learning about others' roles and different ways of doing/seeing things.

Some respondents located their learning in the importance of collaboration for the provision of effective services, by giving examples of settings in which they worked. One person commented that the course reflected aspects of their role in a setting in which there was a range of professional skills and contributions from both health and social services. Another pointed to the fact that interprofessional relationships were a key part of some areas of service provision. Another thought that the course represented the way forward for the delivery of an integrated service. A nurse commented that the interprofessional mix on the course was very beneficial as partnership working was vital in moving forward if you worked in a joint team. Another highlighted the benefit of increased awareness of other professions' agendas, given the need for skill mix, interdisciplinary care plans and assessment.

Perceived drawbacks

Some practice teachers drew attention to perceived drawbacks in relation to the course. One social worker observed that the course had had too broad a focus and had not felt relevant at times. Another commented that on the course the health professionals kept together and so did the social workers. Another felt there had been little benefit as there had only been one non-social work colleague in their particular cohort group (referring to an earlier group before the balance of numbers became more even and perhaps echoing the issue discussed earlier about whether and when a course is *truly* interprofessional). A nurse commented that they felt that the course was predominantly social work oriented. Another person raised the issue as to whether the tutors had had an adequate enough understanding of the other discipline.

The views of managers and training officers

Sixteen questionnaires were returned from managers and training officers who worked in the services from which course participants had been seconded onto the course. The general benefits of the course in terms of professional development were reflected in their responses. All seven managers who responded and seven out of the nine training officers confirmed that the practice teacher's competence in both teaching and practice had increased as a result of undertaking the course. No comments were received from the one training officer who responded negatively to this question.

Positive comments received referred to aspects such as: practice teachers being more objective, keeping up to date with current trends, improved lateral thinking, improved ability to assess the needs of the student, greater consciousness of the learning environment, development of presentation skills and gain in confidence.

Training Officers commented on similar areas, such as the awareness of different perspectives on skill development, increased confidence in practice teaching and the benefit of the practice teacher being better able to support colleagues in the team and not just students.

Respondents were asked about the benefits of their employee being involved in practice teaching and their responses are shown in Table 5.2. These suggest that the majority of participants developed or improved their standard of student supervision and that there was an agreed gain from undertaking interprofessional training. All respondents (n = 16) said they would recommend the course to other employees in the future.

Impact on professional practice

Analysis of the above responses from participants and other stakeholders suggests a number of general professional gains from undertaking this course. This would however, be expected of any well-run practice teacher course. When the managers and training officers list such benefits as greater objectivity, currency of knowledge, lateral thinking and improved presentation skills, it has to be acknowledged they could be commenting on a single professional training course. So what is qualitatively different about an interprofessional one?

We believe that the positive impact upon and relevance to practice of learning these and other skills in an *interprofessional learning environment* is borne out by the evaluation feedback. There are three keys to this:

1   Dialogue – an interprofessional course creates the opportunity for open and honest communication between different professionals. Such a course gives space for dialogue away from the pressures of the workplace. In this space different views, values and cultures meet.
2   Understanding – awareness of the practical aspects of professional roles and responsibilities develops, opening up the possibility

Table 5.2 Benefits of being involved in practice teaching
(16 respondents in total)

	Managers who agreed	Managers who disagreed	Training Officers who agreed	Training Officers who disagreed
Offering placements to students	7	0	9	0
Practice Teaching has increased standard of supervision	5	1	8	0
Practice Teaching has helped to retain staff	6	1	4	2
Practice Teaching has helped staff keep up to date with current trends	7	0	9	0
Links with other agencies	5	2	6	1
Attracted new staff	3	3	6	0
Interprofessional Training	4	2	6	0
Other – enhanced internal communication and work across services			1	

for improved understandings between professionals in practice situations.

3 New Perspectives – critical practice requires practitioners to understand and incorporate new perspectives in relation to their work in a world of practice which is subject to constant change. Learning about and reflecting upon previously unknown perspectives, upon literature about teaching and assessing from other professional

groups, and upon different ways of working lie at the heart of such practice.

An Interprofessional Practice Teaching Course is therefore able to prepare practice teachers not just for the task of practice teaching but also for their own practice in services which are changing, in some cases dramatically, and where roles and professional tasks are being redefined.

Conclusion

Current debates focus on whether interprofessional learning taking place in a university in reality impacts positively on practice and service delivery in health and social care. Interprofessional working is an area of competence already identified in qualifying and post-qualifying courses in health and social care. We would argue that educating *the teachers* in an interprofessional context can offer the opportunity for a cultural challenge by identifying explicitly interprofessional learning opportunities rather than the more traditional focus on offering predominantly uniprofessional experiences (where interprofessional learning opportunities remain unrecognised, implicit or peripheral). This also has the important benefit of reinforcing the requirement for more explicit assessment and evidence of good practice in interprofessional working in the practice element of the *qualifying* courses, which the practice teachers are supporting. As a result of practice teachers' experience of interprofessional learning together and designing and teaching interprofessional learning opportunities, it is hoped that future practitioners will have been provided with more explicit learning opportunities in this area, so enhancing their practice.

Reflection on the experience of developing and delivering the Interprofessional Practice Teaching Course has led us to conclude this chapter with a summary of what we believe has worked during the creative process that this has entailed. We summarise this as follows. What works is:

- An overall balance in different professional groups or less people from a *very wide* range of professional groups.
- The use of a portfolio to provide a variety of evidence with the emphasis on the practice teacher to identify evidence of competency achievement.

- Observation of teaching practice by an experienced practice assessor is essential as it provides the only first hand account of the practice teachers' teaching competency.
- Workshops for practice assessors in order to standardise assessment.
- Tutors from a range of professional backgrounds willing to learn and model interprofessional teaching and learning together.
- Seminar groups with an interprofessional mix alongside opportunities for uni-professional group work and individual tutorial support.
- A Programme Management Committee made up of stakeholders from health and social care services.
- Regular course boards with participants to seek their views on the course process and content.
- Drawing on a range of literature from across professional groups which relates to interprofessional learning and working together, professional values and anti-oppressive practice and adult learning.

Postscript

The course was reviewed by the GSCC in November 2001. It fully met all the professional requirements for social work and was commended for 11 aspects, including interprofessional working, good teaching of anti-oppressive practice and a good system of informal and formal evaluation by participants.

References

Barr, H (2002) *Interprofessional Education Today, Yesterday and Tomorrow* Occasional paper no. 1. Centre for Health Sciences and Practice. Learning and Teaching Support Network.

CCETSW (1996) *Assuring Quality for Practice Teaching.* London: CCETSW.

Bartholemew, A, Davis, J and Weinstein, J (1996) *Interprofessional Education and Training. Developing New Models.* London: CCETSW.

British Association of Social Workers (2002) *The Code of Ethics for Social Work.* Birmingham: BASW.

Cuming, H and Wilkins, H (2000) *Involving Service Users in the Assessment of Students in Professional Practice.* Journal of Practice Teaching, **3**(2), 17–30.

Davis, J, Rendell, P and Sims, D (1999) The Joint Practitioner: A New Concept in Professional Training *Journal of Interprofessional Care* **4**(13).

ENB (2001) *Preparation of Mentors and Teachers. A New Framework of Guidance.* London: ENB/Department of Health.

General Social Care Council (2002) *The Code of Conduct for Social Care Workers* London: GSCC.

Leonard, K (1998) A Process and an Event. The Use of Observation by Practice Assessors and Practice Teachers, chapter in *Observation and its Application to Social Work – Rather like Breathing*. Le Riche, P and Tanner, K (eds) London: Jessica Kingsley.

Nursing and Midwifery Council (2002) *Code of Professional Conduct. Protecting the Public Through Professional Standards*. London: NMC.

Shardlow, S and Doel, M (1996) *Practice Learning and Teaching*. London: Macmillan.

UKCC (1992) *Code of Professional Conduct*. London: UKCC.

Wilmott, S (1995) Professional Values and Interprofessional Dialogue. *Journal of Interprofessional Care,* **9**(3).

6

Interprofessional Post-qualifying Education: Team Leadership

Mike Cook

Chapter overview

This chapter describes a two-year work-based interprofessional Masters Degree Programme, for staff that led teams across London in the health and social care sectors. A framework for health and social care leadership is described and nine leadership themes are identified. A programme based on these nine themes is then presented highlighting issues that the planning team had to consider. One section of the programme is described in more detail, identifying how the programme participants from diverse areas of health and social care worked in an Enquiry Based Learning model to explore aspect of 'vision' in leadership.

The need for improved leadership

Within the literature there has been general agreement that effective leadership is required to achieve high quality care (Booth, 1995; Rowden, 1995; Maggs, 1996; Connolly, 1997; Smith, 1997; Salvage, 1999; Cunningham and Kitson, 2000). *The NHS Plan* (DoH, 2000a) commits the NHS to delivering a radical change programme which requires first-class leaders at all levels of the NHS, who should be 'the brightest and the best of public sector management'. This identified need was additionally highlighted in the strategic plan for London, '*Modernising the NHS in London*' (DoH, 1998) which identified the importance of a well-trained and developed workforce, suitably led and supported. *The NHS Plan* also sets out targets and milestones for modernising the workforce and the health services. Subsequent, documents such as; *A Health Service of All The Talents* (DoH, 2000b) and *Working Together, Learning Together: A Framework for Lifelong Learning* (DoH, 2001a), calls for educators to develop team working among professionals so that staff can be deployed more flexibly, thereby maximising their skills and abilities. For nurses, leadership development was clearly articulated in *Making a Difference: Strengthening the Nursing, Midwifery and Health Visiting Contribution to Health and Healthcare* (DoH, 1999a). For Allied Health Professionals the document *Meeting the Challenge: A Strategy for the Allied Health Professions* (DoH, 2000c) promotes the leadership imperative that 'there is a need to develop leadership skills and capacity more widely among the allied health professions to ensure high quality clinical and managerial leadership' (5.13, p. 38). Whilst less overt about leadership development the Social Service sector expects effective leadership as identified in policy documents such as *Modernising Health and Social Services: Developing the Workforce* (DoH, 1999b) *and Service Quality Improvements in Social Care* (DoH, 2000d). These documents support the view that excellent professional leadership and management capability enhance care provision. This is reinforced in Social Services reports, for example, the following extract from the inspection of service quality improvements in social care Sheffield City Council (DoH, 2000e) 'there was clear leadership from the council and through the Corporate Executive Management Team. The leadership promoted the benchmarking of initiatives with similar councils ... There was much confidence expressed in the leadership of social services from within the council, by staff and by other agencies.'

The need for effective leaders in both the NHS and Social Services is a reflection of Baggotts' (1998) opinion that the environment of healthcare is in constant turmoil, partially due to the lack of agreement as to the strategic priorities. This turmoil has placed significant pressure on staff working in these sectors. This point has been succinctly summarised by Burkitt *et al.* (2000, p. 98) who undertook a study of educational change in care environments 'Pressurised working conditions were something we observed in virtually all workplaces we studied.' It is suggested that the source of these pressures are in part being generated from the following areas:

- the number of elderly people in populations are growing and the proportion of oldest old in particular,

- the number of elderly people living alone is rising (by about 30 per cent since 1948), with a knock-on effect for health and social services,
- the public will continue to expect more involvement in personal health care choices, and in how services were designed and delivered,
- there is a likely decrease in the size of hospitals, with services developing on a more 'local' basis,
- medical technological advances are increasing rapidly with training through virtual reality systems, and 'keyhole' or minimal access surgery,
- pressure on limited resources for public health and social welfare will grow,
- there will be growing pressure on families to provide more social and other forms of support,
- ethical dilemmas such as rationing and euthanasia are becoming more frequently debated and precedents are being determined through the legal system.

This is further impacted upon by a wider changing world which is moving from an industrial age to a quantum age, as portrayed in Table 6.1.

Health care workers and writers have agreed that bureaucratic hierarchies and top down leadership and autocratic management will not be effective in meeting these challenges. The twenty-first century requires speedy responses, coming from flatter, less hierarchical organisations, where roles and jobs are more flexible, with higher and broader skill levels, and greater expectations of close involvement in decision making, from both employer and employee (Porter-O'Grady, 1994; Norman, 1995).

These developments are requiring both the health service and social care to change, and this is leading to a review of the way that people are led and managed. Bolman and Deal (1991, p. 403) state that it is usual for 'leadership to be offered as a solution for most of the problems of ·

Table 6.1 A changing world (influenced by Wheatley, 1994; Capra, 1997)

Industrial age	Quantum age
Linear thinking	Systems thinking
Compartmentalisation	Indistinct boundaries
Process orientated	Outcome orientated
Fixed job requirements	Fluid work requirements
Predictable impacts	Variable impacts

organisations everywhere'. And so it is in health and social care that effective leadership is cited as a major factor that will improve patient care (Cunningham and Whitby, 1997; Cook, 1999; Allen, 2000).

Yet, even with this emphasis on leadership within the NHS signs of leadership failure exist. One report cites high levels of psychological disturbance, ranging from emotional exhaustion to suicide, existed in 29–49 per cent of nurses and that much of this ill health is associated with aspects of work (Williams *et al.*, 1998). Similar figures are reported in the same publication for medical staff and therapists.

Noting this trend of increased ill health amongst health care workers one senior person in the NHS recognised a need for change and called for the introduction of a 'servant leader' ethos amongst those who served the NHS (Jarrold, 1998). Drawing on the work of Greenleaf (1970) Jarrold emphasised trust and integrity, between leaders and teams.

Within the United Kingdom (UK) the Performance and Innovation Unit (Cabinet Office, 2001) undertook a systematic study of leadership in the public sector. The work highlights that there was little shared understanding of the qualities required for effective leadership in today's public services and that there was little evidence as to their effectiveness. It indicated that further investment was required for research into effective preparation for leaders in the public sector and the work was required as to how effective leadership impacted on the service provided, one tentative view was that effective leadership did not necessarily provide the drive for change as generally perceived. This conflicts with evidence from the business sector were robust evidence links effective leadership with improved performance (Joiner, 1994; Dahlgaard *et al.*, 1997). Effective leadership forms a core component of the European Foundation for Quality Management (EFQM) Quality Award. It is therefore suggested that research efforts should now be concentrated on discovering further insights as to how effective leaders use the themes identified in *Embodying Leadership* in the workplace to achieve continuous service improvement.

Definitions

One of the recurring problems when discussing team leadership is that none of the policy documents agree as to what a team or a leader is. Many people seem to be placing the label *team* on any group of people that are working together and an effective leader as the all-controlling 'super-manager'. It is therefore important to define each of these terms.

Teams

The distinction between a group and a team is important. A group is composed of members who are striving to create a shared view of goals and develop an efficient and effective organisational structure on which to accomplish those goals. A group becomes a team when shared goals have been established and effective methods to accomplish those goals are in place (Wheelan, 1999). Whilst different definitions of teams exist the following definition taken from the Indian and Northern affairs, Canada web site (2002) encompasses the main aspects of the various definitions.

A team is a group of people with complementary skills who are committed to a common purpose, performance goals and approach for which they hold themselves mutually accountable and interdependent.

Expanding on these concepts a common purpose allows a team to build an identity, to give itself a direction a momentum. A common purpose gives a team an identity that extends beyond the sum of the individuals involved. A common purpose also ensures stability through change.

Performance goals help a team transform its common purpose into specific and measurable goals.

A common approach enables a team to sort out who will do a particular job, how schedules will be set and monitored, what skills need to be developed, how the group will make decisions, and when and how to modify the approach to ensure successful completion of the teams objectives.

Mutual accountability and interdependence mean that every team member is equally engaged and responsible for accomplishing tasks and achieving goals. These broad areas are reflected in the work of Øvretveit *et al.* (1997) and Thompson and Pickering (2002).

Leadership

Definitions of leadership abound from the great person theory, to the skills attributes stance to the now almost universally accepted contingency view of leadership. The following captures in a very brief but meaningful way the differences between leadership and management, in addition a third role, administration, is introduced as a third leg to the stool of organisational efficiency and effectiveness. Leadership is about path making, doing right things. Management is about path following-doing things right and administration is about path tidying-doing things

(West-Burnham, 1997). Drawing on a previous definition of an effective clinical leader (Cook, 1999), this chapter adopts the following definition of a health or social care team leader 'an expert involved in providing or supporting direct care services who influences others to improve the care they provide continuously'. Unlike many definitions of leadership, this definition does not contain a list of traits, skills or competencies. This definition recognises that effective care requires a cohesive team determined to improve on 'what is', and use influence to achieve this (Sergiovanni, 1992; West-Burnham, 1997). This definition highlights the direct involvement of the leader in developing an effective team.

Background to the programme

Building on national policy the National Health Service Executive, London Region, identified leadership as one of the key themes for workforce development. A leadership-working group was formed in 1999 and devised a project to address the following questions:

*   What kinds of leaders does the NHS require to help plan for, inspire, motivate and lead its workforce?
*   What exactly does a really good leader in the NHS do?
*   What should be done to enable existing NHS leaders to become leaders in a modernised NHS?
*   What should be done to develop new leaders for the NHS?

These questions were put to about 900 leaders, service providers and service users in London's health service and they contributed to generating the meaning of leadership in a modernised NHS (NHSE London, 2000). Results from asking these questions were thematically analysed from which four key themes emerged:

*   More first-class leaders were required to transform the organisation;
*   Leaders should focus on service user needs;
*   Leader development should be through work-based learning;
*   Leaders should ensure cohesion by pulling together strands of work into a coherent whole.

A few quotes from some of the respondents who supported these key themes:

From the centre: *more first-class leaders*

We need clinical and managerial leaders throughout the health service. The best NHS leaders are outstanding. There are simply too few of them. NHS organisations should be led by the brightest and the best ... (DoH NHS Plan, 9.23)

From those responsible for planning: *focus on service user needs*

> At times, I find myself forgetting what made me decide to go into health care in the first place I really would welcome the chance to re-focus on the essentials of matching services with the needs of different groups and communities.

From service providers: *work-based learning*

> I want to capture what I learn at work and have that recognised and validated. We shouldn't always have to go away from the workplace to learn.

From service users and those who care for them: *ensuring cohesion*

> Most of the staff are great – but I don't think anyone is putting it all together. The staff don't seem to be very well looked after themselves.

Using the data enabled the project group to develop a framework for leadership in the NHS in London, based on nine themes:

Articulating a vision
Embodying values
Valuing responsiveness
Encouraging creativity
Developing personal resources
Working across boundaries
Motivation
Taking decisions
Releasing talent.

A short description of each of these themes is provided, further information can be obtained from the *Embodying Leadership* reference at the end of this chapter.

Articulating a vision

Leaders show that they have a clear picture of the world which they aspire to create and build upon. They also have a positive sense of how their vision accords with that of peers and of the organisation as a whole.

Motivation
Leaders show that they care about the people in their organisations by acknowledging them as individuals and by giving recognition for the work that they do and the contributions that they make.

Taking decisions
Leaders are proactive in identifying the decisions that need to be taken and are not afraid of taking them, in situations from the simple to the complex and sensitive. Leaders define the decisions that need to be taken and the criteria that effective decisions need to meet.

Releasing talent
Leaders recognise that *all* people within the organisation, not just the high flyers, have skills, talents or potential to develop and contribute more. They also recognise the value of ensuring that people's talents and skills, once released, are harnessed and not lost to the organisation.

Valuing responsiveness and flexibility
Managing their personal time in a way which allows flexibility and responsiveness. Being able to respond positively and competently to unexpected events. Being able to function effectively in conditions of uncertainty Experiencing change as exhilarating rather than stressful.

Embodying values
Leaders are clear about the values which they hold. By demonstrating their values in their day-to-day actions, they persuade rather than impose their values on others. They view excellence in leadership in a positive light, and as a lynchpin of commitment to public sector values.

Encouraging innovation and creativity
Leaders are constantly striving for better ways to run their organisations and teams, to achieve the goal of delivering highest quality services to their users. They actively encourage people to come up with ideas and suggestions in the common pursuit of this goal, and back new ideas and ways of working. Leaders create a sense of fun and excitement in their organisations.

Working across boundaries
Leaders recognise and acknowledge the complexities within which they work – and are bold in crossing boundaries when that crossing is likely to result in more effective learning and working, more creative solutions and

a better service. They are able to identify tensions that cause problems in working across boundaries and which make innovation difficult.

Developing personal resources
Leaders demonstrate considerable resilience and persistence. When allied to the pursuit of worthwhile goals, these qualities enable leaders to translate vision into reality and to win other people's commitment. They are not easily knocked off course and are able to summon up reserves of energy both to see things through and to handle unanticipated difficulties and problems.

An interesting point to note that whilst these themes have been drawn from a sample of staff working in health care they reflect similar themes found in other work focusing on leadership. For example, the theme of having and conveying a clear vision, of declaring and sharing values and encouraging creativity and motivating others are all clearly stated in the work of Senge (1990) and Senge *et al.* (1994). The work of Drinka and Clark (2000) provides clear links with *Working across boundaries.*

Within the area of initial education head teachers have been required to undertake leadership preparation (Teacher Training Agency, 1998; Male, 2000) and the themes of *Encouraging creativity, Taking decisions and Valuing responsiveness* are evident in School Headship preparation programmes.

The *Embodying Leadership* framework (NHSE, 2000) proved popular, and was put to use in different ways across the health and social care system. The addition of social care to the developing leadership agenda reflected the developing policy papers that identified the need to bring about closer co-operation between health and social care providers (Shifting the Balance of Power, DoH, 2001b). It is interesting to note that despite the framework being developed from a predominantly health care provider population, the Social care sector found value and meaning in the same framework. Recognising the potential for the framework to positively influence health care through development of leaders the NHS Executive London Region commissioned programmes for staff with different leadership responsibilities working in both health and social care. The three different versions of the programme are described below.

Leading Teams is designed for people right at the front end of service delivery – ward sisters/charge nurses, community mental health team leaders, first line managers in support services.

Leading Services is designed for people who have responsibility for shaping whole services, either in a single organisation or across a network such as a cancer network.

Leading Organisations is designed for people who create the organisational climate and culture which enable excellent teams and excellent services to come into being and to be sustained.

Providers for the programmes were secured through a competitive tender process and staff from the Institute of Health Sciences at City University were commissioned to provide the Leading Teams version of the programme. A private consultancy group delivers Leading Services and a charitable organisation delivers the Leading Organisations version.

Using the embodying leadership framework to develop a programme

Founding principles

The programme was developed using the Embodying Leadership framework. A founding principle for the design was to recognise that real leadership does not appear in convenient bite sized chunks, but exists in the 'marshy swamplands' of complex organisations. The *Leadership London* programme was designed to offers clinicians and managers at different levels an opportunity to deepen and extend their expertise as leaders by learning at work. Principles of 'how people learn' (Reynolds *et al.*, 2002) were incorporated and in particular emergent work on work-based learning. This approach has been a major driving force behind the programme design. One of the aims has been to derive a programme that meets of the workplace and of the participant rather than being controlled or framed by the disciplinary or professional curriculum: in the words of Boud and Solomon (2001, p. 5) 'work is the curriculum'. The goal was to support leaders who wanted to transform organisations, modernise services and develop teams. In particular, the programme has two main aims:

- enable leaders to re-create a service which meets the needs of all London's citizens;
- enable participants to gain recognition as professional and competent leaders.

A great deal has been written about leadership and effective teams, yet the impact on actual leadership practice has been less impressive. For services to improve this has to change and it is asserted that this will happen only if leaders are supported, coached and challenged to think and act differently. To prepare leaders to deliver the radical changes outlined in the modernisation policies of the NHS and the Social Services Sector it was considered necessary to re-think aspects of learning and teaching for leadership. The programme designed for staff leading teams, had to be based around the participants' everyday working environment. It was agreed that the nine themes had to be explored in relation to the participant's work and their teams. The programme is proving to be demanding, but participants are being supported to achieve real changes in their everyday work, and so feel inspired to lead the change agenda with increased confidence. The programme through effective facilitation addresses complex issues in interesting and understandable ways, providing carefully designed, learning opportunities that include formal input, web-based activity and paper-based learning materials designed to support participants in their work-based environment.

As stated previously one of the underpinning philosophies was to harness the participants diverse experience, both work and academic. It was therefore considered vital that the programme enabled all participants to share their experiences and learn from each other. The first cohort come from a wide range of NHS and Social Service environments. From within the NHS staff come from, primary care, ambulance trusts, acute hospital trusts, the regional office. They also reflect a mix of disciplines such as: supplies staff, nurses, medics and biochemistry. Social Services staff come from an equally broad base: mental health, older adult and staff that work across both the NHS and social care sectors. Experiences are shared through classroom-based discussions, reflective practice sessions, action learning sets and to a lesser extent web-based materials. It has also been necessary to accommodate a wide range of previous academic experiences. These range from minimal academic experience, to those with higher degrees and doctorates. As the programme team have a great deal of experience of working with students from wide and diverse backgrounds this has not proved to be very problematic.

Selection

To gain a place on the programme each participant completed an application form that asked for general background and details of their experience to date. They also had to complete a short section detailing what they would gain and give to the programme. Applicants had to be supported by their Chief Executive. This was felt to be important as all participants had to have space and time made available to attend all sessions and undertake work-based assignments, this was in addition to

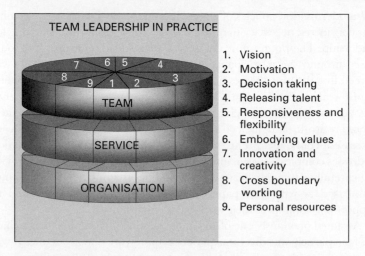

Figure 6.1   Integrated programme structure

guaranteeing web access and a contribution to book purchases, course fees were paid by the Workforce Development confederation, who supported the programme. It can therefore be seen that the London Region were investing heavily in this programme.

Figure 6.1 shows the three levels and nine themes as an integrated whole. Work has been ongoing with each of the partners to ensure that the programme remains integrated, and opportunities for learning from both different sectors and between people at different levels of the organisations in which they work.

Programme aims and outcomes?

The broad aims of this programme were to develop healthcare personnel who were able to:

- deal with complex issues both systematically and creatively, make informed judgements in the absence of complete data and communicate their conclusions clearly to specialist and non-specialist audiences;
- demonstrate self-direction and originality in tackling and solving problems and act autonomously in planning and implementing tasks at a professional or equivalent level;

- continue to advance their knowledge and understanding, and to develop new skills to a high level.

The following outcomes reflect the abilities that a typical participant completing the programme will be able to demonstrate:

- Able to understand and work in the turbulent climate of healthcare and, regardless of their position in the organisation, be able to work effectively in partnership across the boundaries of disciplines and levels.
- Be able to demonstrate a willingness to experiment and innovate in order to develop and improve practice and clinical care.
- Be committed to creating supportive environments to enable change to occur.
- Become skilled in leading, managing and developing interprofessional and inter-agency collaboration.
- Be able to access and critically evaluate evidence of the social and political context in which health care is delivered and strategically contribute to developing those services.

Facilitating the participants to achieve the course outcomes whilst undertaking demanding jobs

The following principles were devised to ensure that the programme remained focused, coherent and meaningful to participants:

- the programme uses real world learning opportunities, drawn from action leaning sets.
- participants at each of the three levels; organisation, service and team have opportunities to work with and learn from each other.
- participants work with different professional groups at different levels of the organisation.
- The participants have opportunities to spend time outside of the NHS and Social Services working in different but equally complex organisations.

How is the programme working in practice?

Figure 6.2 provides the programme outline demonstrating how participants have the option of completing the Masters programme in two years, whilst others might wish to 'step-off' the course having completed

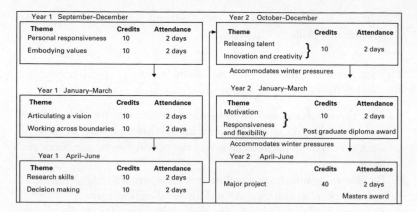

Figure 6.2 Programme outline

the nine themes and would receive a post graduate diploma. Other participants might not present their work for formal assessment, but complete the course and have a record of work-based improvement and the development of personal skills, attributes and behaviours.

At a more detailed level the first two days of learning enables the programme participants to share their leadership learning to date through a range of carefully constructed activities, using a range of leadership assessment tools (psychometric tests, interviews, work samples, simulated group decision-making exercises) coupled with 'real world' thinking. These were designed to prepare them for working as a group and ready to share their strengths and weaknesses. Additionally they were introduced to action learning sets, portfolio development and reflective thinking.

The programme has three other 'attendance' days where it is intended that they work with and share learning with members of their own health care community from the other two versions of the programme; services and organisations. The plan is to facilitate them to tackle a specific improvement project as a team, in close co-operation with service users, their representative and informal cares. For logistical reasons this is still proving problematic to implement, but it is believed that the benefits will be significant and work is progressing to achieve this aspect of the programme. Close co-operation between all partners exists and is helping programme compatibility.

Workshops are an additional feature of the programme and whilst yet to be delivered are intended as an opportunity for participants to identify some possible areas of special interest to them such as:

Inclusivity and the diversity agenda
Confident presentations
Handling the media
Factors the facilitate and constrain effective leadership
Networking and collaborating
Lobbying skills.

How is learning being assessed?

It was agreed that the major purpose of the assessment was to act as an aid to improving leadership in the workplace. This means that participants are exposed to a variety of assessment modes. To date these have been well received, although not without problems. For instance one of the modules required the participants to present their Enquiry Based Learning findings, the presentation was assessed, with a team mark being awarded. All groups demonstrated outstanding skills, yet one group received a lower grade for their work. This proved to be very contentious and is requiring the planning team to reconsider this approach. Participants are expected to maintain a reflective diary to provide a learning log of changes to their workplace and leadership practice. For some participants this is relatively straightforward having been exposed to this learning approach previously. For others it is proving to be a significant learning challenge as they have not previously been encouraged to state their feelings and document their personal learning using any reflective practice. The design and delivery team are learning that the needs of participants varies significantly and a further learning point has been to build significant academic support into the programme. All participants do not require this but for those that do it can be time consuming.

The major project to be assessed for the Masters award has to demonstrate rigour and achievement of Masters level work. This may be an 8000-word dissertation or an alternative piece of work negotiated with the programme team. This might, for example, take the form of a piece of work directly related to the participants work environment, and may result in a significant report, a video tape or computer software or perhaps development of training material.

Assessment criteria

Each assessment has clear criteria, broadly these include assessment of:

- the project purpose, aim and objectives;
- impact on the workplace;

- evidence of original thinking;
- evidence of cognitive skills, application, analyses and evaluation;
- integration of theories and principles from relevant disciplines;
- critical evaluation of research and literature.

Dedicated web site

Participants have access to a number of electronic support features on a dedicated web site, this includes bulletin boards, chat rooms and email access. It is possible for students to send material for uploading to the web site. Various links are available to other leadership web sites, including the National Nursing Leadership site, to ensure best use of these developing resources, and to encourage collaborative networking across the NHS and social care sector. It was planned that access to the web site would be integral to learning, yet it is interesting to note that few of the team version participants are using the web site to any great extent. Reasons for this are part of an ongoing evaluation of the programme.

Support from other experienced leaders

Each participant has access to a personal tutor. The personal tutors hold posts in either the NHS or Social Services. Where possible, the participant will retain them for the duration of the programme to provide support and guidance. The following guidelines have been agreed as a guiding framework.

- Facilitating unblocking impasses in the work setting.
- Helping with action planning, time management (both work and study) including milestones and targets.
- Helping prioritise work/study issues in times of work pressure.
- Providing help with the 'bigger picture'! A wider view of policy and practice locally, nationally and, where appropriate, internationally.
- Enabling the application of theory to practice.
- Facilitating networking and advancing the personal and professional development of their participant partner. In particular providing support to those in minority positions in their workplace role.
- Modelling awareness of and demonstrating ways of challenging institutional racism and sexism within the NHS.
- Ensuring time is set aside exclusively for participants and being 'on their side' in ways which are both supportive and challenging.
- Assist in the development of the Portfolio (where relevant).

It was considered important that the personal tutor should not be the participants line manager and where possible they have been drawn from another discipline.

To clarify expectations and to agree and evaluate the role, academic staff and the personal tutors meet together on a regular basis. As well as providing participant support, some personal tutors are using the partnership as an opportunity for personal growth and development.

A unit of learning described

To provide more insight into the programme design one of the programme modules is outlined to show how learning from experience is achieved. The main educational emphasis was to enable the participants to think differently and this meant moving away from teaching them to providing tools that led to new ways of thinking.

The module described has the title *Articulating the Vision*. The module aimed to enable participants to critically analyse the importance of generating a vision that aligns with and meets organisational imperatives. To place the responsibility for learning with the participant in this module Enquiry Based Learning (Glen and Wilkie, 2000) was utilised. None of the participants had used EBL before, so this also provided an opportunity for them to experience a mode of learning that appears to be growing in popularity within the health services. In this way they would become familiar with techniques being used by the students they were supervising in practice.

The learning outcomes of the module were:

1 Critically assess the impact of leadership principles and values on the workforce and the development of healthcare practice.
2 Critically evaluate the purpose of visions in organisations, explore suitable alternatives to vision and mission statements.
3 Critically evaluate the critical features of a meaningful vision for organisations and their realisation.
4 Draw on organisational theories to identify key features of a personal vision.
5 Drawing on relevant literature show how people can be engaged in developing and making a vision tangible.

The content for this module was based around the following indicative topic headings.

- Investigating organisations
- Organizational change theories
- Vision and mission in organisations
- Learning organisations
- Collaboration and independence
- Accountability and reward
- Personality theory
- Following others.

The participants were spilt into four groups of seven to eight people and two facilitators led the groups. The participants had one three hour facilitated session to plan their work, and further support was available if requested. Each group undertook the work differently, some met for meetings and progress updates before the presentation. Others used electronic communication to plot progress and plan work; one group did neither but planned their individual work quite carefully before leaving the first facilitated session. A few weeks later they presented their findings, which were assessed as a group with an individually written supporting 'article' reflecting on their experience and identifying how the learning would impact on their practice in the workplace. It was interesting that all groups presented some form of role play; a method that at the start of the programme they had resisted with specific requests not to have to do any role-play. Each group agreed to work on one scenario. One of the groups engaged with the following scenario:

> Your team has received well-deserved recognition for implementing a new service. The service helps to ensure effective discharge from acute care services for people with long-term health needs. You have been seconded from your team to implement the same service across London. You have one year to set up the service and have minimal resources at your disposal. The launch of this new service, 'soon to be available' across London is highly publicised, with significant political support. You are asked to outline your plans for the future to a NHSE steering group. You commence the presentation to a group of interested faces.

The scenario was designed to enable to participants to draw on their own experiences, it was known that many had implemented new services and others were required to implement new services in the near future. In this way the group had an opportunity to share their experiences and to have their own ideas explored by people with different experiences. It was anticipated that this scenario would draw on some of the agreed attributes of effective leaders. For instance with respect to creativity this activity provided some space for creative thinking. Buzan (2000) and Senge (1990) both highlight the importance of creating special space and time for creative thinking. In addition the ability to maintain a flow of information enables creativity. Having access to information helps people to consider alternative courses of action. It was anticipated that the aspect of respecting others would be explored as the group become more sensitive to signals from others within their group and learn about signals that were organisationally based.

One of the key aspects that this scenario was designed to draw out was the team leader's ability to 'influence' others. This is a well-recognised attribute of effective leaders. In this scenario the participants had the opportunity to explore their ideas about how they would influence decision makers to back their ideas. The scenario was designed to encourage participants to consider their vision of the project. Drawing on the work of Covey (1999) and Senge (1990) the participants were encouraged to consider the end point of their change project and to see how by aligning their own objectives with that of the wider organisation, support from influential stakeholders would be more likely to be forthcoming. The scenario also drew out the support that both themselves and their team required. They also identified the importance of setting up suitable support networks for their own and their teams development.

Discussion and conclusions

One of the most demanding aspects of the programme development from a curriculum design aspect has been developing close co-operative working between the providers of the service and organisation version of the programme. Additionally for the providers of the service and organisation versions a further university provider is involved in aspects of accrediting their work-based learning. To ensure that the Team version provided by City University has parity with these other versions close collaboration is required. In addition to this already complex arena, close working is required with the commissioning body the Work Force Development Confederations across London. This complex developmental scenario is achieved through a *virtual faculty* consisting of all parties and student representation. Whilst initially it took some time to adapt to this way of working it is now proving both stimulating, new ideas are generated quickly, and I believe enhancing the experience of those undertaking the programme. A word of caution to anyone else pursuing similar shared initiatives is to ensure that a shared framework of standards for quality assurance is developed. Whilst the learning has to benefit the organisation the programme leads to a formal academic award and as such has to meet rigorous quality standards.

Given the complexity of the leadership role it was difficult at times to tease out elements of each of the nine individual themes. Delivering the programme has demonstrated that overlaps between themes are occurring naturally. The participants are making these links for themselves as demonstrated in discussion and their assignments. By having opportunities to learn together, through projects of their own design, the participants are recognising that others have similar issues to address and are sharing positive ways of dealing with difficult problems.

Through close liaison between all the programme providers it should be possible to generate opportunities for participants from all three versions to work together in 'health and social care communities', on specific care improvement projects. This has always been a desire amongst the programme providers, but is still proving problematic to actualise. On reflection it should have been considered earlier in the programme design and perhaps might be achieved with closer liaison between each of the providers.

The Action Learning Sets have been contentious as not all participants find this mode of learning particularly helpful. Four action-learning sets were set up with experienced facilitators for each one. Three are operating well and appear to be meeting the participants needs. One is problematic and whilst a simple diagnosis is not encouraged for complex learning groups, and respecting the confidentiality of the group, it appears that amongst other things the group would rather spend the time allocated to other more conventional forms of independent study. The fact that all groups are interprofessional suggests that this is not a root of the cause. It is suggested that course planners for similar programmes explore with participants their preferred learning styles and try to accommodate these as far as possible.

The uptake of the support offered by the Personal Tutors has varied considerably between participants. Some made swift contact and have developed productive and meaningful relationships, sharing work related issues and concerns. Others have had minimal, or no contact and this has not necessarily been a lack of availability of the personal tutor. It seems that some participants prefer not to use this source of support. For some personal tutors that offered their time and support, this has been disappointing for them as they were keen to be supportive. It seems that some of the participants prefer to work in a more individual way, which makes on wonder about how they are working with their own teams.

For some reason the participants of the Team programme are not using the web site extensively at all. Further work is ongoing to identify why this might be the case, although it is has been suggested that the schedule of the working day does not allow time for access, study time is too precious to surf for what might be useful. When they have very specific material to gather it is known that many of the participants are email active and communice between themselves using this medium.

Overall the time and energy invested in developing this work-based Interprofessional Team Leadership programme is proving worthwhile. The interprofessional learning appears to be significant and whilst the current cohort are yet to complete, early evaluations suggest that the focus of work-based learning is having beneficial effects on the participants, their teams and more importantly the users of their services.

References

Allen, D (2000) The NHS is in Need of Strong Leadership. *Nursing Standard*, **14**(25), 25.

Baggott, R (1998) *Health and Health Care in Britain* (2nd edn). London: Macmillan Press.

Bolman, L G and Deal, T E (1991) *Reframing Organisations; Artistry Choice, and Leadership*. San Francisco: Jossey Bass Publishers.

Booth, B (1995) Leading Frights ... Effective Leaders. *Nursing Times*, **91**(23), 58.

Boud, D and Solomon, N (2001) *Work-based Learning: A New Higher Education?* Buckingham: The Society for Research into Higher Education and Open University Press.

Burkitt, I, Husband, C, Mackenzie, J, Torn, A and Crow, A (2000) Evaluating Cognitive and Affective Processes in Educational Preparation for Individualised Care in Pre and Post registration Education and Practice; Final Report to the ENB., Ethnicity and Social Policy Research Unit, University of Bradford.

Buzan, T (2000) *Head First: 10 Ways to Tap into Your Natural Genius*. London: Thorsons.

Cabinet Office, Performance and Innovations Unit (2001) *Strengthening Leadership in the Public Sector: A Research Study by the PIU*. London: Cabinet Office. http://www.cabinet-office.gov.uk/innovation/leadershipreport/piu-leadership. pdf (accessed 31/01/02).

Capra, F (1997) *The Web of Life*. London: Harper Collins, Flamingo.

Connolly, M (1997) The Naked Truth ... Nursing Leadership. *Nursing Times*, **93**(12), 27.

Cook, M J (1999) Improving Care Requires Leadership in Nursing. *Nurse Education To-day*, **19**(4), 306–12.

Covey, S R (1999) *The 7 Habits of Highly Effective People, Powerful Lessons in Personal Change*. London: Simon & Schuster Ltd.

Cunningham, G and Kitson, A (2000) An Evaluation of the RCN Clinical Leadership Development Programme: Part 2. *Nursing Standard,* **15**(13–15), 34–40.

Cunningham, G and Whitby, E (1997) Power Redistribution, *Health Management,* September, 14–15.

Dahlgaard, J J, Larsen, H Z, Norgaard, A (1997) Leadership Profiles in Quality Management. *Total Quality Management,* **8**(2,3), 516–30.

Department of Health (1998) *Modernising the Health Services in London – a Strategic Review.* London: Department of Health.

Department of Health (1999a) *Making a Difference: Strengthening the Nursing, Midwifery and Health Visiting Contribution to Health and Healthcare.* London: Department of Health.

Department of Health (1999b) *Modernising Health and Social Services: Developing the Workforce.* London: Department of Health.

Department of Health (2000a) *The NHS Plan A Plan for investment A Plan for Reform.* London: Department of Health.

Department of Health (2000b) *A Health Service of All The Talents.* London: Department of Health.

Department of Health (2000c) *Meeting the Challenge: A Strategy for the Allied Health Professions.* London: Department of Health.

Department of Health (2000d) *Service Quality Improvements in Social Care.* London: Department of Health.

Department of Health (2000e) *Inspection of Service Quality Improvements in Social Care.* London: Sheffield City Council, Department of Health.

Department of Health (2001a) *Working Together, Learning Together: A Framework for Lifelong Learning.* London: Department of Health.

Department of Health (2001b) *Shifting the Balance of Power: Securing Delivery.* London: Department of Health.

Drinka, T J K and Clark, P G (2000) *Health Care Teamwork: Interdisciplinary Practice and Teaching.* Westport, CT: Auburn House.

European Foundation for Quality Management web site (see http://www.efqm. org/new_website (accessed 18/10/02).

Glen, S and Wilkie, K (2000) *Problem-based Learning in Nursing.* London: Macmillan Press.

Greenleaf, R K (1970) *The Servant as Leader.* Cambridge, MA: Centre for Applied Studies.

Indian And Northern Affairs, Canada (2002) Leadership and Learning Guide: Teams Handbook, http://www.ainc-inac.gc.ca/ai/ldr/tc_e.html (accessed June 2002).

Jarrold, K (1998) A View from here 'Servants and Leaders'. In Martin, S (ed.) *The York Symposium on Health, 30 July.* University of York: Department of Health Studies.

Joiner, B L (1994) *Fourth Generation Management: The New Business Consciousness.* New York: McGraw Hill.

Maggs, C (1996) Debate, Professors of Nursing as Clinicians and Academics: Is this the Way Forward? *Nt Research*, **1**(2), 157–8.

Male, T (2000) LPSH: Some Observations and Comments. *Management in Education*, **14** (2), 6–8.

NHSE, Workforce and Development Leadership Working Group (2000) *Workforce and Development: Embodying Leadership in the NHS.* London: Department of Health.

Norman, A (1995) Professional Leadership in Community Nursing Services. *Health Visitor*, **8**(1), 21–3.

Øvretveit, J, Mathias, P and Thompson, T (1997) *Interprofessional Working for Health and Social Care.* London: Macmillan Press.

Porter-O'Grady, T (1994) Whole Systems Shared Governance: Creating the Seamless Organisation. *Nursing Economics*, **12**(4), 187–95.

Reynolds, J, Caley, I and Mason, R (2002) *How do People Learn?* Research Report. London: Chartered Institute of Personnel and Development.

Rowden, R (1995) Crisis? What Crisis? ... There is No Evidence that Nursing Lacks Potential Leaders as the Profession has No Shortage of Inspiring and Able People. *Nursing Times*, **91**(37), 50.

Salvage, J (1999) Speaking out ... Supersisters ... Clinical Leadership. *Nursing Times*, **95**(21), 22.

Senge, P (1990) *The Fifth Discipline The Art and Practice of the Learning Organization.* London: Doubleday.

Senge, P, Ross, R, Smith, B, Roberts, C and Klener, A (1994) *The Fifth Disciple Fieldbook.* London: Nicholas Brearley Publishing.

Sergiovanni, T J (1992) *Moral Leadership; Getting to the Heart of School Improvement.* San Francisco: Jossey-Bass.

Smith, S (1997) The Loneliness of a Long-term Leader ... . The 12th National Ward Leaders' Conference in London on May 7 and 8. *Nursing Times*, **93**(12), 30–1.

Teacher Training Agency (1998) Leadership Programmes for Serving Headteachers: Handbook for Participants. London Teacher Training Agency.

Thompson, J and Pickering, S (2002) Developing a Culture for Change. In Howkins, E and Thronton, C (eds) *Managing and Leading Innovation in Health Care.* London: Harcourt, 185–210.

West-Burnham, J (1997) Leadership for Learning – Reengineering 'Mind Sets'. *School Leadership and Management*, **17**(2), 231–44.

Wheatley, M (1994) *Leadership and the New Science: Learning about Organisations from an Orderly Universe.* San Francisco: Berrett-Koehler Publishers.

Wheelan, S A (1999) *Creating Effective Teams: A Guide for Members and Leaders.* Thousand Oaks CA: Sage.

Williams, S, Michie, S and Pattani, S (1998) Improving the Health of the Workforce. *Report on the Partnership on the Health of the NHS Workforce.* London: the Nuffield Trust.

7

Interprofessional Education: The Evidence Base

Sally Glen

Introduction

Evaluation is a characteristic that has developed in advanced capitalist society (House, 1993). The belief that institutions and culture can be deliberately fashioned through experimentation and research is one of the hallmarks of twentieth century and early twenty-first-century thought (Norris, 1990). A major theme that has been at the heart of the debate about evaluation, since it emerged as a substantial field of activity, is the role of evaluators in relation to policy making and policy makers. In 1982 Cronbach suggested that a modest aspiration for evaluation was to contribute to decision making as policy development in the long term (Simons, 1987). Due to the challenges of interprofessional education; the logistics of bringing students together; the curriculum changes required; the efforts of staff and students to be expanded and the upheaval of health and social care institutions to facilitate contact. In addition to the mixed messages about the ultimate goals of interprofessional education coming from various public and professional bodies (cf. Chapter 1), it is essential the move is evidence-based, and contributes to ongoing policy development in this area. As Kendall and Lissaur (2003) note:

> A key barrier to interprofessional training is the lack of evidence about it's effectiveness. More investment in evaluating interprofessional learning must be provided in future. [xv]

However, the relationship between interprofessional education evaluators to policy making and policy makers is not clear.

Establishing the evidence base

The ability of health professionals to work together collaboratively is critical to delivering patient-centred care. The proposition that learning together may help people to work together more effectively is thus intuitively reasonable. However, this immediately leads to more difficult questions about:

- For what kind of interprofessional learning experiences should one aim?
- What are the outcomes of interprofessional education?
- How can the impact of interprofessional education be detected?

In the context of the prevailing 'evidence-based' agendas the need to provide empirical support for the effectiveness of interprofessional education is increasing. Evaluations seem to be most sure-footed in capturing students' experience and weighing implications for programme modifications; less so in establishing the impact of learning on practice, still less benefit to service users (Barr *et al.*, 1999 and CAIPE/DOH, 2002). Very few studies provide evidence of longer-term outcomes, in particular on professional practice. Positive outcomes from university-based interprofessional education typically meets interim objects, for example: student satisfaction, changes in knowledge and attitude and, occasionally, individual behaviour. However, studies available are all largely atheoretical, based on short-term interprofessional inputs and have used outcome measures which address short-term effects only, often immediately post intervention.

Research into the effects of interprofessional education is beginning to identify a favourable range of outcomes associated with this activity. These include the enhancing of teamwork skills and improving the knowledge of different professional roles (Barr, 2002). Evidence to date also suggests that the greater integration of interprofessional education into the wider curriculum the more positive the effect on attitudes to interprofessional collaborative working (Barnes *et al.*, 2000; Horsburgh *et al.*, 2001). Freeth *et al.*, 2002 grouped the reported outcomes of inter-professional education into six categories: learners' reactions, changes in attitude or perception, changes in knowledge or skill, behavioural changes, changes in the organisation or delivery of care, benefit to patients or clients. Freeth *et al.* (2002) suggest that:

- Around 90 per cent of interprofessional education occurs in the United States.
- Most interprofessional education courses (60 per cent) have a duration of over two weeks.
- Interprofessional education tends to be evaluated by relatively 'weak' designs (e.g., before-and-after and post-intervention designs).
- Practice-based interprofessional education that has a duration of over two weeks tends to report a positive impact on clients and patients (e.g., reducing length of hospital stays, client/patient satisfaction).
- Practice-based interprofessional education appears to have more impact on clients and patients in acute rather than chronic care settings.

There is a stronger culture of evaluation of social programmes, including education, in the United States (US) than in, for example, the UK. While the following characterisation may be slightly overdrawn, it draws attention to the social embeddedness of theories and models of evaluation:

> Mechanistic analogies have a peculiar appeal for people who see themselves as the raw materials of a vision which can be socially engineered. Their culture is characteristically forward looking, constructionist, optimistic and rational. Both the vision and the optimism are reflected in the assumptions that goal consensus, a pre-requisite of engineering, is a matter of clarification rather than reconciliation. In contrast, British culture is nostalgic, conservationist, complacent and distrustful of rationality …. MacDonald in Hamilton (1977)

However, if expectations and the allocation of funding discourage the sound evaluation of interprofessional education, education policy makers and providers will continue to make decisions from a relatively weaker evidence base. Alternatively, they will be reliant upon evidence from a context which may have a different value system and which operates in different social and political contexts. In the UK, greater investment is needed in evaluating interprofessional learning, across the spectrum of contexts. Such evaluations would contribute to our knowledge about the place and role of interprofessional education in professional curricula. These evaluations will also provide valuable evidence about effective curricula design and inform educators about how to maximise learning outcomes, in addition to informing policy developers.

All educational innovators should operate a plan-do-study-act cycle to ensure high quality, well-targeted provision. What is required is:

- A small number of comprehensive evaluations of different types of interprofessional education.
- Evaluation of innovation, in the pedagogy and evaluation of interprofessional education.
- Prospective studies with lengthy follow-up periods.

Evidence of this nature will ensure that the interprofessional education practice of the future is informed by robust evidence for effectiveness across the wide range of provision.

Work-based interprofessional education

Preliminary evaluation suggests that practice-based interprofessional education is much more likely than university-based education to impact positively on clients and patients. Learning and exposure to good role models in practice has long been recognised as being more influential than learning and role models within higher education institutions. The aims of interprofessional work-based education might therefore be to:

- Provide students with an understanding of the roles, cultures and values of different professions leading to benefits for clients and patients.
- Develop greater confidence among students by addressing the issue of 'professional protectionism' and identifying the usefulness of an overlap in roles, which is different from wasteful duplication.
- Secure a more cost-effective way of providing education and training.
- Contribute to a learning culture that fosters reflection, analysis and evaluation by focusing on interactive learning.

It is generally accepted that adult learning is more likely to be effective if it is interactive and problem – case – or task-focused. The workplace provides an ideal setting for health and social care professionals to develop and practice interprofessional collaboration skills, especially when the placements are in service settings, where different professionals are involved in providing care (Freeth *et al.*, 2001). An effective working relationship between higher education institutions (HEIs) and service organisations is fundamental to the development of interprofessional work-based education. Workforce Development Confederations must work with universities to develop appropriate work-based learning. This should be supported through a system of fair reward for staff who support work-based learning, linked to incentives, appraisal and performance assessment (Humphris and Macleod Clark, 2002).

Conclusion

It is vital that research investment is identified and directed towards this policy area (Zwarenstein *et al.*, 2000). Interprofessional education needs to develop new models of interprofessional learning and teaching and demonstrates improvements in: education, professional practice and patient and client care. It also needs to document improvements in health status and health and social care services. In addition, interprofessional education needs to address questions such as: does the integration and collaboration in improvement efforts accelerate improvement and accentuate benefits to participants, students, faculty members, health and social care organisations and patients, carers and users? Does the learning and teaching process accelerate the pace of change and learning in existing educational programmes. We must also not loose sight of uni-professional education and strengthening individuals' contribution to the team providing care.

We need more interpretative and critical studies. Although expensive and relatively difficult to publish, there is much to be gained from qualitative studies. Since most interprofessional education initiatives are multifaceted, a greater number of mixed method studies would be advantageous. It is comparatively difficult to secure funding for qualitative or mixed methods research studies of education interventions for health and social care. There is much to be gained from addressing the multifaceted resistance to such studies. However, Humphris and Macleod Clark (2002) make the following cautionary note:

> The 'evidence-based' dilemma that will be faced in the promulgation of interprofessional learning, as with all innovation, is that of change to the existing order. The dilemma simply put is that without innovation evidence cannot be developed. Yet the mantra of the 'evidence-base' could potentially become a constraint to the innovation necessary to address the significant workforce challenges faced by the future of health and social care.

Evaluation, in some conception, is an attempt to use the authority of science to legitimate and inform government actions in societies in which the traditional institutions have lost much of their legitimating power. Given the current Government's investment in interprofessional education one might also argue evaluation will be required to legitimate this policy directive – as noted in Chapter 1, interprofessional education has become managerially driven, resistance has become politically unacceptable.

References

Barnes, D, Carpenter, J and Dickenson, C (2000) Interprofessional Education for Community Mental Health: Attitudes to Community Care and Professional Steroetypes. *Social Work Education,* **19**(6), 565–83.

Barr, H (2002) *Interprofessional Education Today, Yesterday and Tomorrow: A Review.* London: LTSN Hs & P.

Barr, H, Hammick, M, Koppel, I and Reeves, S (1999) Evaluating Interprofessional Education: Two Systematic Reviews for Health and Social Care. *British Educational Research Journal,* **25**(4), 533–43.

Centre for the Advancement of Interprofessional Education (CAIPE)/ Department of Health (2002). Selected case studies of interprofessional education. CAIPE/DOH 2002.

Cronbach, L J (1982) *Designing Evaluation of Educational and Social Programs.* San Francisco, CA: Jossey Bass.

Freeth, D, Reeves, S and Goreham, C (2001) 'Real Life' Clinical Learning or an Interprofessional Training Ward. Sustaining Inter-Professional Collaboration, *Journal of Inter-Professional Care,* **15** (1), 37–46.

Freeth, D, Hammick, M, Koppel, I, Reeves, S and Barr, H (2002) A Critical Review of Evaluations of Interprofessional Education. London: Centre for Health Sciences and Practice, Learning and Teaching Support Network.

Hamilton, D (1977) Making Sense of Curriculum Evaluation: Continuities and Discontinuities in an Educational Idea, University of Glasgow. In Sulman, L (ed.) *Review of Research in Education,* **5**, Itasca, IL: Peacock Press, 318–47.

Horsburgh, M, Lamdin, R and Williamson, E (2001) Multiprofessional Learning: The Attitudes of Medical, Nursing and Pharmacy Students to Shared Learning. *Medical Education,* **35**, 876–83.

House, E R (1993) *Professional Evaluation: Social Impact and Political Consequences.* Berkeley Hills, CA: Sage Publications.

Humphris, D and Macleod Clark, J (2002) *Shaping a Vision for a 'New Generation' Workforce.* Southampton: University of Southampton.

Kendall, L and Lissaur, R (2003) *The Future Health Worker.* London: Institute of Policy, Practice and Research.

Norris, N (1990) *Understanding Educational Evaluation.* London: Kogan Page Ltd.

Simons, H (1987) *Getting to Know Schools in a Democracy: The Politics and Process of Evaluation.* Lewes: Falmer Press.

Zwarenstein, M, Reeves, S, Barr, H, Hammick, M, Koppel, I and Atkins, J (2000) *Interprofessional Education: Effects on Professional Practice and Healthcare Outcomes* (Protocol for a Cochrane Review). Oxford: The Cochrane Library.

Index

action learning sets   80, 92, 98
Annandale, E   19

Baggott, R   80
Barnes, D   18, 21
Barr, H   5–6
Blackfriars Centre   63
Bolman, L G   81
Boud, D   55, 88
Bristol Inquiry   2–3
Bristol Royal Infirmary   2
British Association of Social Workers
    Code of Ethics   67
BSc (Hons) modules   57
BSc in Nursing and Social Work studies
    (Learning Difficulties)   64
Burkitt, I   80
Burrows, D E   26
Bury, M   18
Buzan, T   97

CAIPE *see* Centre for the Advancement of
    Interprofessional Education
Care Planning Approach   16
Centre for the Advancement of
    Interprofessional Education (CAIPE)
    5, 8, 65
Chamberlain, J   23
City University programme   58
Civil Emergency Management   49
Clark, P G   87
CMHNs *see* Community Mental Health
    Nurses
CMHTs *see* Community Mental Health
    Teams
Code of Conduct
    for nurses   67
    for social care workers and social care
        employers   67

College of Occupational Therapy   62, 64
Commission for Health
    Improvement   24
'common' studies *see* 'core' studies
community care   7, 17
Community Mental Health Nurses
    (CMHNS)   20
community mental health teams (CMHTs)
    xv, 29–44
    work-based interprofessional education
        for   29–44
Community Nursing Programme   64
content delivery   53–5
Continuing Professional Development
    framework   56
Cook, M   xvi, 79
'core' studies   12
Course Advisory Board   48–9
course developers   8, 54
Course Management Team   48–9
course validation document   69
Covey, S R   97
Cronbach, C J   102
Cuming, H   70
Curriculum Management Team   49

data analysis   34
data collection
    follow-up interviews   33
    observations   33
    questionnaires   33
Deal, T E   81
Department of Adult Nursing   49
Department of Health   3, 23
    policy emphasis   3
Diploma in Social Work (DipSW)
    programme   63
Doel, M   70
Drinka, T J K   87
Dubyan, J   21

108

(EBL) *see* Enquiry-Based Learning
educational facilitation 26
education and training 17, 20–3, 25–6
Edwards, K 18
EFQM *see* European Foundation for
    Quality Management
Embodying Leadership 82, 85, 87
    framework 88–91
Emergency Care Practitioners 2
Enquiry-Based Learning (EBL) xvi, 54,
    79, 95
    model 79
European Declaration of Human
    Rights 46
European Foundation for
    Quality Management (EFQM) 82
evaluation 102–4, 106
    programme 57
    social embeddedness of theories and
        models of 104
    of the workshops 32
evidence base, establishing the 103–6

feedback 49, 57, 64, 69, 71, 74
    from course participants 71
Fenge, A L 24
Finch, J 6
Forrest, S 17
Foundation Degrees 2
Freeth, D 103–4

General Social Care Council (GSCC)
    65, 68
Glen, S 1, 102
group and a team distinction
    between 83
GSCC *see* General Social Care Council

Hanson, B 17
healthcare
    personnel 90–1
    policy 1
    practice 95
    practitioners 2–3
    teams 2
Health Improvement Plans xv, 1

higher education institutions (HEIs) 2,
    11–12, 105
Hopton, J 19
Human Rights 46–7, 53
Humphris, D 106

Insituto de Psicologia Applicada in
    Lisbon, Portugal 47
interprofessional collaboration 5, 105
interprofessional course xii, 9, 58, 65–6,
    68, 74
interprofessional education xi–xii, xvii,
    1, 9, 30–1, 65, 69, 102, 106
    definitions 65
    delivering the workshops 31–2
    educational factors 9
    evidence base 102–7
    policy context 1–15
    and practice 45–60
    project development 31
interprofessional initiatives 10–11
interprofessional learning 12, 99
Interprofessional Master of Science
    Programme xvi, 46
interprofessional Masters Degree
    Programme 79
interprofessional post-qualifying
    education 61, 79
    team leadership 79–101
    and training 16
    user and carer involvement in 16–28
interprofessional practice 45
    development of a Masters
        Programme 45
    MSc 51
interprofessional practice teacher
    education 61–78
Interprofessional Practice Teaching
    Course 61, 63–4, 76
    background and development 63–4
    opportunity to learn 64
Interprofessional Team Leadership
    programme 99

Joint Practice Teaching Initiative
    (JPTI) 62
Jose Ornelas, Prof. 47

Kendall, L   102
Kings Fund   24
Koppel, I   30, 51, 57

Labour Government   xv, 1, 4
leadership
    based on nine themes   85–8
    definitions of   83
    improving in the workplace   93
    need for improved   79–82
Leadership London programme   88
Lee Ann Hoff, Dr   47
Leiba, T   xv, 16
Leonard, K   xvi, 61, 70
Lissaur, R   102

MA in Social Work   64
Macleod Clark, J   106
managers
    views of   73
Masters programmes   52, 56, 91
    course structure   52
    modules   52
Mental Health Foundation   24
mental health and social care
    professionals   25
Metropolitan Police Service   48
Miller, C   5, 7
Mitchell, D   17
modernisation policies of the
    NHS   89
modernising the workforce   9, 80
MSc programme   49, 51, 53, 57
Multi-Agency Public Protection
    Panels   47

National Health Service (NHS)   1–7, 11,
    17, 19, 65, 70–1, 79–80, 82, 84–5,
    87, 89, 91, 94, 96, 99
National Health Service Executive,
    London Region   84
National Nursing Leadership site   94
National Service Frameworks   xv,
    1, 24

Nottingham University   20
Nursing and Midwifery Council
    (NMC)   64

Obholzer, A   48

palliative care   7, 22
Patients Charter   19
Performance and Innovation Unit   82
personal tutors   57, 94, 96, 98
Pirrie, A   9
post-workshop perspective   38
practice
    assessor   69–70, 77
    teachers   61–2, 71–2, 75
    tutorials   70
pre-workshop perspective   35
professional practice   74
Programme Management Committee
    (PMC)   65
Pryce, A   10
Public Health Practitioners   2

Quinn, C   21

Raine, P   23
Reeves, S   xv, 10, 29–30
Reflective Practice sessions   53, 55, 89
Research Assessment Exercise   23
Roberts, V Z   57
Rogers, J A   23

Sainsbury Centre   17–18
Sally, G   xv–xvi
Schon, D   xii, 22
School of Nursing and Midwifery   56
Senge, P   87, 97
Shardlow, S   70
Shields, P   18
Simpson, A   20–1
Sims, D   xvi, 61
socialization   3, 8, 10
Social Services Sector   89
Solomon, N   88
South Bank Practice Teaching
    Programme   63

South Bank University   61
Sully, P   xvi, 45
'super-manager'   82

team
  leadership   82
  learning experience   39
  programme   99
training officers   xvi, 41, 71, 73–4
  views of   73
Truman, C   23
Turner, P   22

uniprofessional education   6, 66, 76
user involvement in research   23–5

violence   xiii, xvi, 45–9, 51–4, 56–8
  extent and consequence of   xvi

web site   83, 94, 99
Wilkins, H   70
Wilmott, S   67
Wilson-Barnett, J   17, 19
Wood, J   17, 19
work-based interprofessional education
  105–6
Workforce Development Confederations
  12, 90, 97, 105
Working Time Directive   xv, 1
workshops   xv, 22–3, 29, 31–42,
  49, 53, 57, 77, 92–3
  content of   32
  delivering   31
  during   36
  experiences   38
World Health Organisation's
  report   58